Rheumatology
Continuing Education Review

407 Essay Questions and Referenced Answers in Rheumatology

By

ANTHONY BOHAN, M.D.
Clinical Assistant Professor of Medicine
University of California
Irvine Medical Center
Orange, California

Staff Rheumatologist
Hoag Memorial Presbyterian Hospital
Newport Beach, California

Co-Director
Orange County Arthritis Medical Group, Inc.
Orange, California

Medical Examination Publishing Co., Inc.
an Excerpta Medica company

969 Stewart Avenue/Garden City, New York 11530

Copyright © 1978 by
MEDICAL EXAMINATION
PUBLISHING CO. , INC.
an Excerpta Medica company

Library of Congress Card Number
78-62494

ISBN 0-87488-333-4

September, 1978

Printed in the United States of America

PREFACE

The field of rheumatology has been one of the most rapidly expanding areas of medicine in the past several years. New concepts and techniques have been developed, and old ones discarded. Entirely new illnesses and syndromes have appeared, which five or six years ago did not exist. Therefore, one major objective of this review has been to summarize, in a comprehensive fashion, these important newer developments, both in the clinical as well as in the laboratory context.

Another important objective has been to review, in a broad manner, the basic concepts inherent in studies of rheumatic, arthritic, and connective tissue disorders.

This treatise, therefore, may be useful in a number of directions. For the physician preparing for the National Boards or the State Boards, for Flex, or for the specialty examinations in internal medicine, family medicine, orthopedic surgery, pathology, and other related disciplines, this book will bring together the basic concepts, as well as the recent advances, in a brief but authoritative manner. For the rheumatologist or clinical immunologist preparing to take the sub-specialty examination in rheumatology, this survey will prove helpful in reviewing fundamentals, emphasizing the important developments in the recent rheumatological and immunological literature, and detecting areas where further study would be prudent.

As is true of any brief survey of a broad and complex field, no attempt can be made to thoroughly encompass the whole of the subject matter. Therefore, the physician utilizing this book should think of it as a guide to the basic rheumatological and immunological literature, as referenced in the questions.

For the physician who is not preparing for an examination, but who wishes to stay abreast of developments in this field, or who would like to gain a better perspective in the area of rheumatic disorders, this book will provide him with a sweeping panorama of the subject matter but with sufficient detail for a practical application to everyday clinical problems.

Although some unusual and rare conditions have been included in this volume, the emphasis is not on esoterica but instead is on the fundamentals of rheumatic diseases, both old and new.

Anthony Bohan, M.D.

RHEUMATOLOGY
Continuing Education Review

CONTENTS

I. RHEUMATOID ARTHRITIS

1. Q. What are the most useful parameters in the assessment of rheumatoid activity?

A. Perhaps the most accurate parameter as to activity in rheumatoid arthritis is the patient's own assessment of the severity of pain. Other parameters which appear to reflect disease activity in patients with rheumatoid arthritis are the synovial fluid polymorph count, synovial fluid glucose estimation, and serum C-reactive protein estimation.

REF: Farr, M. , Kendall, M. J. , Young, D. W. , et. al. "Assessment of rheumatoid activity based on clinical features and blood and synovial fluid analysis." Ann Rheu Dis 35:163-167, 1976.

2. Q. Discuss the role of synovectomy of the knee joint in rheumatoid arthritis.

A. Early synovectomy of the knee in rheumatoid arthritis appears to be effective in reducing pain and locally controlling inflammation in 69% of patients. Preservation of articular cartilage was noted in 71%. However, a relatively large recurrence rate is present in up to 28% of cases with progressive loss of cartilage and persistent inflammatory synovitis. The optimum time to perform synovectomy is in the instance when medical therapy has failed to control inflammation and when there is still no evidence of damage to the articular cartilage.

REF: Ranawat, C. and Desai, K. "Role of early synovectomy of the knee joint in rheumatoid arthritis." Arth Rheum 18:2, 117-121, 1975.

3. Q. Describe the elements of the rheumatoid hyperviscosity syndrome.

A. The hyperviscosity syndrome in rheumatoid arthritis is relatively rare and has been reported infrequently. Clinically, patients generally present with nodular rheumatoid arthritis, weakness, dyspnea, a generalized bleeding diathesis, and a striking red palmar erythema. In the laboratory, high titers of rheumatoid factor are present with large amounts of intermediate IgG immune complexes. Serum viscosity measurements indicate that the very high serum viscosity is due to the interaction of the rheumatoid factor with the intermediate IgG complexes.

REF: Jasin, H. E., LoSpalluto, J., and Ziff, M. "Rheumatoid Hyperviscosity Syndrome." Am J Med 49, 484-493, 1970.

4. Q. What are the types of pulmonary lesions seen in rheumatoid arthritis?

A. The most common manifestation is perhaps that of pleurisy with or without pleural effusion. In addition, Caplan's syndrome may be seen which consists of a rheumatoid pneumoconiosis. Pulmonary rheumatoid nodules, diffuse interstitial pulmonary fibrosis and interstitial pneumonitis may occur. An unusual type of pulmonary involvement is that of the intima of the small pulmonary arterioles resulting in pulmonary hypertension.

REF: Walker, W. C. and Wright, V. "Pulmonary lesions and rheumatoid arthritis." Medicine 47:6, 501-520, 1968.

5. Q. Discuss the general concepts of rheumatoid hand deformities.

A. The major factors involved in the development of the various rheumatoid hand deformities are as follows: (1) Improper adaptation to normal stresses by inflamed or weakened supporting structures; (2) abnormal stresses that are the result of muscle imbalance and mechanical alterations. These stresses are all dynamically induced. Treatment and prevention of these deformities would therefore involve vigorous control of joint inflammation, physical measures designed to promote range of motion, the minimization of joint stress, and when necessary, early surgical correction of existing deformities.

REF: Swezey, R. L. "Dynamic factors in deformity of the rheumatoid arthritic hand." Bull Rheum Dis 22:1, 2, 649-656, 1971.

6. Q. Discuss the clinical setting in which one might expect to find decreased serum complement levels in rheumatoid arthritis.

A. Although serum complement levels are generally either normal or increased in rheumatoid arthritis, in rare instances a significant decrease in the serum complement may be seen. This observation has been made in patients with severe rheumatoid arthritis associated with marked destruction, and multiple extra-articular complications such as vasculitis or rheumatoid pleuritis. A positive correlation is seen between hypocomplementemia and subcutaneous nodules, positive rheumatoid factor tests, and greater functional impairment.

REF: Franco, A. E. and Schur, P. H. "Hypocomplementemia in rheumatoid arthritis." Arthritis and Rheum 14:2, 231-238, 1971.

7. Q. Discuss the frequency and significance of cerebrovascular and coronary artery disease in rheumatoid arthritis.

A. In patients with rheumatoid arthritis, the frequency of myocardial infarction in terms of morbidity and mortality is significantly less than expected. However, no differences were noted between the frequency of coronary artery atherosclerosis, cerebral infarction or pulmonary embolization. These findings have been interpreted to mean that there may be a lesser incidence of thrombosis, perhaps due to the inhibition of platelet aggregation by salicylate therapy.

REF: Davis, R. F. and Engleman, E. G. "Incidence of myocardial infarction in patients with rheumatoid arthritis." Arthritis and Rheum 17:5, 527-533, 1974.

8. Q. What are the features of "rheumatoid nodulosis?"

A. Rheumatoid nodulosis is considered to be an unusual variant of rheumatoid arthritis. Multiple subcutaneous nodules are present throughout the hands and feet. In addition, multiple cystic radiolucencies are noted throughout bones of the hands, wrists, and feet.

REF: Ginsberg, M. H., Genant, H. K., Yu, Tsai F., and McCarty, D. J. "Rheumatoid nodulosis." Arthritis and Rheum 18:1, 49-57, 1975.

9. Q. Discuss the complication of esophageal varices in connection with Felty's Syndrome in rheumatoid arthritis.

A. Felty's syndrome is the combination of splenomegaly, leukopenia, and rheumatoid arthritis. Extra-articular manifestations are common. These may include mild liver function abnormalities, portal hypertension, esophageal varices, and recurrent upper gastrointestinal hemorrhage. In a patient with Felty's syndrome, the presence of portal hypertension with varices and gastrointestinal bleeding may thus serve as another indication for splenectomy.

REF: Klofkorn, R. W., Steigerwald, J. C., Mills, D. M., and Smyth, C. J. "Esophageal varices in Felty's syndrome." Arth Rheum 19:1, 150-154, 1976.

10. Q. What is the role of chronic salicylate therapy in liver function tests in juvenile rheumatoid arthritis?

A. High serum salicylate levels above 30mgm% may produce elevation of the serum transaminases, as well as alkaline phosphatase abnormalities and occasional prothrombin time prolongation. However, liver function abnormalities may also occur during periods of low serum salicylate levels, and a precise statistical correlation between serum salicylate levels and transaminase elevation is lacking. Chronic hepatotoxicity has been noted in patients on long-term salicylate therapy.

REF: Miller, J. J. and Weissman, D. B. Arth Rheum 19:1, 115-118, 1976.

11. Q. What is the relationship between cigarette smoking, obstructive pulmonary disease, and rheumatoid arthritis?

A. Smokers with rheumatoid arthritis had a significantly increased frequency of obstructive pulmonary disease than did smokers with degenerative joint disease or non-smokers with rheumatoid arthritis. In a study of 43 patients, 60.5% of these patients who were cigarette smokers and who fit the ARA criteria for classical rheumatoid arthritis were found to have significant obstructive pulmonary disease. There may be the possibility therefore that the combination of tobacco smoking and rheumatoid arthritis facilitates the development of obstructive pulmonary disease.

REF: Collins, R. L., Turner, R. A., Johnson, A. M., et. al. Arth Rheum 19:3, 623-628, 1976.

12. Q. Discuss the effect of pregnancy on the course of rheumatoid arthritis and some of the theoretical considerations that may underlie this observation.

A. In general, patients with active rheumatoid arthritis improve during pregnancy and relapse again following delivery. However, not all patients with rheumatoid arthritis improve, and perhaps 25% of patients may experience either no improvement or actual worsening during the period of gestation. A variety of potential factors that could account for these observations has been considered. These include placental extracts, "acute phase" proteins such as fibrinolysis and coagulation proteins, and pregnancy zone protein (PZP). The latter has been studied in considerable detail. It is found in low concentrations in nonpregnant women, increases during gestation in most but not in all women, and decreases again following delivery. It appears to be a stabilizer of lysozomal membranes, and in addition has several effects on T-cell function. These observations may explain in part the variable improvement that is observed clinically in pregnant women with rheumatoid arthritis.

REF: Persellin, R. H. "The effect of pregnancy on rheumatoid arthritis." Bull Rheum Dis 27:9, 922-927, 1976-1977.

13. Q. What is the diagnostic specificity of skin basement membrane immunofluorescence in patients with rheumatoid arthritis and positive lupus serology?

A. Skin biopsy material from patients with rheumatoid arthritis is consistently negative for immunofluorescence along the basement membrane. This observation holds for rheumatoid patients with positive lupus serology such as a positive lupus cell preparation or positive anti-nuclear antibody titer. This of course is in contrast to patients with systemic lupus erythematosus wherein positive basement membrane immunofluorescence is commonly seen in both involved as well as uninvolved skin.

REF: DeBoer, D.C., Moskowitz, R.W., Michel, B. Arth Rheum 20:2, 653-656, 1977.

14. Q. Discuss the coagulation abnormalities in patients with rheumatoid arthritis and rheumatoid vasculitis.

A. Plasma fibrinogen levels are known to be elevated in patients with rheumatoid arthritis, whether or not vasculitis is present. However, in patients with vasculitis, the fibrinogen, platelet count and fibrin splint products tend to be elevated more frequently than in uncomplicated rheumatoid arthritis. Active plasmin may also be detected in patients with vasculitis. These results may be interpreted as demonstrating overcompensated intravascular coagulation and fibrinolysis that appears in rheumatoid vasculitis.

REF: Conn, D.L., McDuffie, F.C., Kazmier, F.J. et.al. "Coagulation abnormalities in rheumatoid disease." Arth Rheum 19:6, 1237-1242, 1976.

15. Q. What are the earliest radiographic abnormalities to appear in rheumatoid arthritis?

A. The typical marginal erosion is an early sign of rheumatoid arthritis. In nearly 90% of patients followed prospectively, erosive changes occurred within the first two years following the onset of rheumatoid disease. Changes in the feet were more commonly seen than in the hands. Osteoporosis is also an early manifestation that may proceed rapidly in the first three years. Joint space narrowing, which indicates irreparable joint damage, occurred within the first two years in 49% of the patients with erosive disease.

REF: Brook, A. and Corbett, M. "Radiographic changes in early rheumatoid disease." Ann Rheum Dis 36, 71-73, 1977.

16 . Q. What are the features of Brown's syndrome?

A. Brown's syndrome is an unusual manifestation of rheumatoid arthritis. The syndrome is described as including vertical diplopia, a clicking sensation, and an apparent inferior oblique palsy. It is believed that the mechanism causing this syndrome is a stenosing tenosynovitis of the superior oblique tendon and its sheath.

REF: Killian, P.J., McClain, B., and Lawless, O.J. "Brown's syndrome." Arth Rheum 20:5, 1080-1084, 1977.

17. Q. Compare and contrast the development of scleritis and corneal ulcerations in a patient with rheumatoid arthritis.

A. Scleritis, when it occurs in adult rheumatoid arthritic patients, is generally seen in patients with severe arthritis, with evidence of erosive disease, positive rheumatoid factors, nodules, and extra-articular manifestations, especially vasculitis. On the other hand, patients who develop corneal ulceration generally have relatively inactive rheumatoid arthritis, without the tendency for extra articular manifestations, and often with negative rheumatoid factors.

REF: Jayson, M.I.V. and Easty, D.L. "Ulceration of the cornea in rheumatoid arthritis." Ann Rheum Dis 36, 428-432, 1977.

18. Q. Discuss the present concepts of delayed hypersensitivity in rheumatoid arthritis.

A. Although certain functions of cellular immunity have been found to be normal by some investigators, in general, most studies of delayed hypersensitivity in rheumatoid arthritis have described various abnormalities in lymphocyte functions. Skin test reactivity has been found to diminish with increasing rheumatoid activity. Both peripheral and synovial lymphocytic responsiveness has been reduced in patients with extensive disease. Although lymphocyte responses defined by blastogenesis or production of lymphokines have been generally reduced, mixed lymphocyte responses have been either reduced or normal, and occasionally even enhanced. Enumeration of T and B cells has yielded inconsistent results in the peripheral circulation, whereas synovial lymphocytes have now been demonstrated to be predominantly T lymphocytes.

REF: Lloyd, T. M. , and Panush, R. S. "Cell mediated immunity in rheumatoid arthritis." J Rheum 4:3, 231-144, 1977.

19. Q. Describe the present concepts of classification of the various subgroups in juvenile rheumatoid arthritis.

A. Three distinct subgroups have been delineated in JRA. The first subgroup is that of systemic JRA characterized by the presence of fever, polyarticular joint symptoms, skin rash, anemia, leukocytosis, and other extra-articular manifestations. This is the most serious type of JRA. The second group constitutes children with polyarticular disease who have infrequent extra-articular manifestations, and in whom fever, skin rash, anemia, and leukocytosis are much less commonly seen than in the former group. The third subgroup in JRA is that of pauciarticular disease referring to involvement of less than five joints. The course is generally benign, and there appears to be little evidence of erosive or crippling arthritis.

REF: Brewer, E. J. , Bass, J. , Baum, J. , et. al. "Current proposed revision of JRA criteria. JRA Criteria Subcommittee of the Diagnostic and Therapeutic Criteria Committee of the American Rheumatism Association Section of The Arthritis Foundation." Arth Rheum (suppl) 20:195-199, 1977.

20. Q. Comment on the association of antinuclear antibodies, immune complexes, and clinical manifestations in juvenile rheumatoid arthritis.

A. Antinuclear antibodies are most often found in pauciarticular juvenile rheumatoid arthritis. They are therefore also associated with chronic iridocyclitis. Immune complexes are generally absent in these patients. However, in the systemic form of JRA, immune complexes were seen more frequently and appeared to be correlated somewhat with severity of disease and systemic manifestations.

REF: Rossen, R.D., Brewer, E.J., Person, D.A., et.al. "Circulating immune complexes and antinuclear antibodies in juvenile rheumatoid arthritis." Arth Rheum 20:8, 1485-1490, 1977.

21. Q. Discuss the current concepts of cervical discovertebral involvement in rheumatoid arthritis.

A. Rheumatoid arthritis not infrequently affects the cervical spine. The diarthrodial joints are synovial joints and it is therefore not surprising that these joints are commonly affected. The discovertebral joints, which are fibrocartilaginous joints such as the sternomanubrial joint or the symphysis pubis, are usually spared. The traditional explanation given for this frequent discovertebral involvement in the cervical spine has been the idea that rheumatoid inflammation of the disc occurs, perhaps from nearby neurocentral joints. However, a somewhat more plausible hypothesis is that this discovertebral destruction is induced by repetitive microtrauma as a consequence of cervical instability, apophyseal arthritis, laxity of ligamentous and supporting structures, and subluxations of the cervical vertebrae.

REF: Martel, W. "Pathogenesis of cervical discovertebral destruction in rheumatoid arthritis." Arth Rheum 20:6, 1217-1225, 1977.

22. Q. Describe the effect of thoracic duct drainage in rheumatoid arthritis and the implications as to pathogenesis.

A. In patients with severe rheumatoid arthritis undergoing thoracic duct lymphocyte drainage procedures, grip strength, ring size, duration of morning stiffness, and the number of tender joints all appeared to improve during the procedure. Reinfusion of autologous lymphocytes appeared to correlate with transient exacerbation of the rheumatoid arthritis. When thoracic duct drainage was discontinued, repopulation of lymphocytes was accompanied by clinical exacerbation of arthritis. However, the arthritis was often

somewhat more easily managed by various antiinflammatory agents. Although both T and B lymphocyte functions
were affected by lymphocyte drainage, it appeared that delayed hypersensitivity (T cell function) was somewhat more
impaired.

REF: Paulus, H. E. , Machleder, H. I. , Levine, S. , et. al.
Arth Rheum 20:6, 1249-1262, 1977.

23. Q. Free DNA may be found in the serum of rheumatoid arthritic patients. Comment on the significance of
this observation and on the clinical correlates as to disease
activity.

A. In a fairly large proportion of patients with rheumatoid arthritis, significant levels of free DNA may be
measured in the serum. These levels are frequently highest in patients with severe rheumatoid disease, and in patients who have had persistent and active rheumatoid synovitis for less than ten years. Patients with less active
disease, or who have had chronic and long standing arthritis, were less likely to demonstrate free DNA levels of
high degree. It has been hypothesized that early in the
course of an inflammatory process, there is easier access
to the circulation of various intracellular components such
as DNA. Later in the disease, these components would be
removed from the circulation by antibodies forming antigen
antibody complexes which would then be phagocytized, dis-
rupting lyosozomal membranes, and releasing enzymatic
material capable of perpetuating the cycle by altering
further nuclear material.

REF: Leon, S. A. , Ehrlich, G. E. Shapiro, B. , and
Labbate, V. A. "Free DNA in the serum of rheumatoid
arthritis patients." J Rheum 4:2, 139-143, 1977.

24. Q. In skin biopsy direct immunofluorescence of unaffected skin, compare and contrast the findings in rheumatoid
arthritis and systemic lupus erythematosus.

A. In systemic lupus erythematosus, there is evidence
of granular deposition at the dermal-epidermal junction of
IgG, IgM, complement components, and components of the
alternate pathway. However, in rheumatoid arthritis, these

immunoglobulins and complement components are characteristically absent from the dermal-epidermal junction. Instead, localization of these elements may be found in dermal vessels from unaffected skin of the leg. It has been hypothesized that these deposits may be correlated with rheumatoid vasculitis, which is known to affect the lower limbs in preference to the upper extremities.

REF: Schroeter, A. L., Conn, D. L., and Jordon, R. E. "Immunoglobulin and complement deposition in skin of rheumatoid arthritis and systemic lupus erythematosus." Ann Rheum Dis 35, 321-325, 1976.

25. Q. In a child with severe rheumatoid degeneration of the hip but who otherwise is in a state of relative remission as far as arthritic involvement of other joints is concerned, comment on the advisability of total hip replacement.

A. Although hip pain may be severe and functional limitations excessive, total hip joint replacement is generally contraindicated in children because of the small size of the hip joint and the potential for further growth. In a report of 6 children with advanced rheumatoid hip disease, it was further noted that with vigorous physiotherapy and emphasis on weight bearing, some bone remodeling may result in clinical and radiographic improvement with partial restoration of the hip.

REF: Bernstein, B., Forrester, D., Singsen, B., et. al. "Hip joint restoration in juvenile rheumatoid arthritis." Arth Rheum 20:5, 1099-1104, 1977.

26. Q. Discuss HLA tissue typing in rheumatoid arthritis.

A. Unlike ankylosing spondylitis and Reiter's syndrome, there is no increased frequency of the antigen HLA B27 in rheumatoid arthritis. However, the frequency of HLA Dw4 has been noted in 36% of rheumatoid arthritic patients as opposed to 13% in controls. The relative risk for a Dw4 positive individual for developing rheumatoid arthritis is estimated at 3.0. An association with Cw3 has also been noted, but is felt to be due to linkage disequilibrium for this allele with Dw4.

REF: McMichael, A. J., Sasazuki, T., McDevitt, H. O., and Payne, R. O. "Increased frequency of HLA Cw3 and HLA Dw4 in rheumatoid arthritis." <u>Arth Rheum</u> 20:5, 1037-1042, 1977.

27. Q. What is the significance of histidine in rheumatoid arthritis and comment on the clinical trials performed with L-Histidine in the treatment of this disorder.

A. There has been convincing evidence that the concentration of histidine in the serum of patients with active rheumatoid arthritis is decreased. Although the cause of this hypohistidinemia is unknown, this fact has stimulated speculation that treatment with histidine may lead to clinical improvement. Several studies have addressed themselves to this issue with conflicting results. In an earlier study, significant clinical improvement was described. However, in a more recent study with placebo controls, no objective improvement by the conventional parameters was forthcoming. It has been concluded that further evaluation will be necessary before any conclusions can be drawn.

REF: Pinals, R. S., Harris, E. D., Burnett, J. B., and Gerber, D. A. "Treatment of rheumatoid arthritis with L-Histidine: a randomized placebo controlled, double blind trial." <u>J Rheum</u> 4:4, 414-419, 1978.

28. Q. Offer a clinical definition of classical rheumatoid arthritis.

A. Rheumatoid arthritis is a chronic symmetrical, polyarthritis with features that suggest a systemic disorder lasting more than six weeks. Multiple joints are involved, and this usually is considered to be at least three, but often four, five, six, and more. The disease is typically symmetrical, both as to right and left symmetry, as well as symmetry around the joint itself. The term "arthritis" of course refers to the presence of articular swelling, heat and erythema. Systemic features include the well known morning gel phenomenon, fatigue, subcutaneous nodules, weight loss, and the other well known extra-articular manifestations associated with rheumatoid arthritis.

REF: Boyle, J. A. and Buchanan, W. W. "Clinical Rheumatology." Blackwell Scientific Publications, Oxford and Edinburgh, 1971, p. 96-166.

29. Q. Describe the clinical and laboratory features of procainamide-induced lupus erythematosus.

A. The most commonly observed clinical features are polyarthralgia, myalgia, recurrent fever, and pleuritic chest pain. Renal involvement is typically absent. The laboratory features are similar to those of naturally occurring lupus with the exception that complement is usually normal and antibody to native DNA is either absent or found in low titer.

REF: Blomgren, S. E., Condemi, J. J., and Vaughan, J. H. "Procainamide-induced lupus erythematosus." Am J Med 52, 338-348, 1972.

30. Q. What are the various types of visual disturbances that may occur in systemic lupus erythematosus?

A. When systemic lupus erythematosus involves the central nervous system, cerebral vasculitis may result in the following features. Out of 12 patients studied, five underwent detailed evaluation for hallucinations which were either unformed or detailed. Four patients had visual loss including scotomas, homonymous field defects, and cortical blindness. Additional findings associated with visual disturbances often included vocal cord paralysis, diminished gag reflex and other findings suggesting posterior cerebral dysfunction. Three patients appeared to have a combination of visual disturbances that included hallucinations and loss of vision.

REF: Brandt, K. D., Lessell, S., Cohen, A. S. "Cerebral disorders of vision in systemic lupus erythematosus." Ann Intern Med 83: 163-169, 1975.

31. Q. Discuss the typical antinuclear antibody "profiles" in systemic lupus erythematosus, rheumatoid arthritis, Sjogren's syndrome, progressive systemic sclerosis, dermatomyositis, and mixed connective tissue diseases.

A. The Sm-antigen, which is an acidic nuclear protein, is generally quite specific for systemic lupus erythematosus

and is rarely found in other rheumatic diseases. The anti-
native DNA titer is frequently elevated to high levels in lupus, whereas its titer in various other rheumatic disorders
such as rheumatoid arthritis, dermatomyositis, Sjogren's
syndrome, and progressive systemic sclerosis is either
negative or only mildly elevated. Antibody to nuclear ribonucleoprotein is found in nearly all cases of mixed connective tissue disease, but may also be elevated in other
systemic rheumatic diseases as well.

REF: Notman, D. D., Kurata, N., and Tan, E. M. "Profiles of antinuclear antibodies in systemic rheumatic
diseases." Ann Intern Med 83:464-469, 1975.

32. Q. Discuss the clinical course and survival rate in systemic lupus erythematosus comparing and contrasting patients with renal involvement and patients without renal
disease.

A. In a study of 30 patients characterized by renal
biopsy as either having significant renal involvement or not,
and followed for an average of 9. 4 years, it was noted that
53% of the "renal" group and 70% of the "non-renal" group
had died. The major factor in the "non-renal" group was
the emergence of cerebral lupus which eventually occurred
in 100% of the "non-renal" group patients. It was noted that
after 8.3 years, the mortality in the "non-renal" group ex-
ceeded that in the renal group.

REF: Cheatum, D. E., Hurd, E. R., Strunk, S. W., and
Ziff, M. "Renal histology and clinical course of systemic
lupus erythematosus." Arth Rheum 16:5, 670-676, 1973.

33. Q. Comment on the use of corticosteroid medication
and immunosuppressive drugs in combination in the treatment of systemic lupus erythematosus and renal disease
due to lupus nephritis.

A. There is as yet no clear consensus on the treatment of lupus nephritis. Corticosteroid medication is the
mainstay of treatment. When corticosteroid medication is
combined with immunosuppressive drugs, additive therapeutic benefit has been claimed by some and denied by others.
There is little doubt, however, regarding the toxicity of these

agents and all agree that they should be used with great caution and with strict adherence to protocol. Two recent clinical trials with combination corticosteroid and immunosuppressive medication failed to demonstrate a significant advantage over corticosteroid drugs alone.

REF: (1) Donadio, J. V., Holley, K. E., Wagoner, R. D., et. al. "Further observations on the treatment of lupus nephritis with prednisone and combined prednisone and azathioprine." Arth Rheum 17:5, 573-581, 1974.
(2) Decker, J. L., Klippel, J. H., Plotz, P. H. and Steinberg, A. D. "Cyclophosphamide or azathioprine in lupus glomerulonephritis." Ann Intern Med 83:606-615, 1975.

34. Q. Discuss the features of transverse myelopathy in systemic lupus erythematosus.

A. In general, the diagnosis of transverse myelopathy is difficult to establish as being due to systemic lupus erythematosus, with the diagnosis being made in only 60% of cases before the onset of the neurological involvement. The most typical presenting feature was either numbness or weakness of the legs or both. Marked reduction of the cerebrospinal glucose was noted. The role of corticosteroid medication has been uncertain, although more favorable results seem to occur when treatment is initiated early. The prognosis is dismal in most cases with death or permanent neurological deficit virtually inevitable in nearly all cases.

REF: Andrianakos, A. A., Duffy, J., Suzuki, M., and Sharp, J. T. "Transverse myelopathy in systemic lupus erythematosus." Ann Intern Med 83:616-624, 1975.

35. Q. Discuss the frequency of serological and hematological abnormalities that are seen in chronic discoid lupus erythematosus.

A. In chronic discoid lupus without evidence of systemic involvement, the frequency with which laboratory abnormalities are seen is quite low. In a study of 80 patients, the following data were noted: anemia (2%), reduced total complement (4%), reduced C3 (8%), positive anti-nuclear antibody (4%), biological false positive VDRL (3%), positive rheumatoid factor (1%), immunofluorescence of normal skin (0%); there were no patients with positive lupus cell preparations, anti-nDNA titers, or lymphocytotoxic autoantibodies.

REF: Prystowsky, S.D., Herndon, J.H.Jr., and Gilliam, J.N. "Chronic cutaneous lupus erythematosus (DLE)." Medicine 55:2, 183-191, 1975.

36. Q. What are the most reliable parameters with which to determine the prognosis in lupus nephritis?

A. Patients with lupus nephritis are best followed by sequential C3 measurements as well as by DNA-binding titers. These parameters provide more sensitive measures of renal disease and may serve as earlier indicators of renal involvement than measurement of the protein excretion or creatinine clearance. In those patients in whom serial renal biopsy has been performed, the complete dissolution of subendothelial deposits was found to be the most reliable histological factor in determining a favorable outcome.

REF: Hecht, B., Siegel, N., Adler, M., et.al. "Prognostic indices in lupus nephritis." Medicine 55:2, 162-181, 1975.

37. Q. Discuss the incidence of infection in systemic lupus erythematosus.

A. In a comparison of lupus patients with rheumatoid arthritic patients and with patients demonstrating idiopathic nephrotic syndrome, data suggested a significantly increased incidence of various infections in the lupus population. Although lupus patients on corticosteroid medication and with decreasing renal function were found to have more frequent infections, a significant increase in the infection rate was also noted for lupus patients with normal renal function and on low dose corticosteroid medication. These data suggest that patients with systemic lupus erythematosus are prone to infectious complications.

REF: Staples, P.J., Gerding, D.N., Decker, J.L., and Gordon, R.S., Jr. "Incidence of infection in systemic lupus erythematosus." Arth Rheum 17:1, 1-10, 1974.

38. Q. Discuss the frequency and the proposed pathogenetic mechanisms of ischemic bone necrosis in systemic lupus erythematosus.

A. Most patients with systemic lupus erythematosus who develop ischemic necrosis of bone are on corticosteroid medication. Multiple bone lesions are frequently seen (83%). The most common sites of involvement are the femoral heads (91%), humeral heads, and tibial plateaus. Raynaud's phenomenon (61%) and central nervous system involvement (43%) are noteworthy in this group of lupus patients. Thus in 87% of patients, some form of vascular involvement could be demonstrated either in the form of Raynaud's phenomenon or systemic vasculitis. It is felt that the microcirculation is thus affected in lupus by either vasospasm or by vasculitis resulting in ischemic lesions in the bone.

REF: Klipper, A.R., Stevens, M.B., Zizic, T.M., and Hungerford, D.S. "Ischemic necrosis of bone in systemic lupus erythematosus." Medicine 55:3, 251-257, 1976.

39. Q. Discuss the diagnostic criteria proposed for systemic lupus erythematosus and the relative sensitivity and specificity of these criteria.

A. The preliminary criteria for the classification of systemic lupus erythematosus are as follows: facial erythema, discoid lupus, Raynaud's phenomenon, alopecia, photosensitivity, oral or nasopharyngeal ulceration, arthritis without deformity, LE cells, chronic false positive STS, profuse proteinuria, cellular casts, pleurisy or pericarditis, psychosis or convulsions, hemolytic anemia, leukopenia, or thrombocytopenia. When applied to groups of patients, a sensitivity of 88% can be expected as compared to a specificity of 97.5% against rheumatoid arthritis patients. If the antinuclear antibody titer is substituted for the lupus cell preparation, sensitivity is increased to 92% without sacrificing specificity.

REF: Trimble, R.B., Townes, A.S. Robinson, H., et. al. "Preliminary criteria for the classification of systemic lupus erythematosus (SLE)." Arth Rheum 17:2, 184-188, 1974.

40. Q. What is the role of the fourth component of complement in the cerebrospinal fluid of patients with lupus cerebritis?

A. When serial determinations of the fourth component of complement are made in patients with systemic lupus erythematosus who develop either acute neurologic or psychiatric syndromes due to lupus cerebritis, then a depression of titer is noted at the time of acute central nervous system involvement. It has been suggested, therefore, that these data support the concept of immune injury in the pathogenesis of lupus central nervous system disease.

REF: Hadler, N.M., Gerwin, R.D., Frank, M.M., et. al. "The fourth component of complement in the cerebrospinal fluid in systemic lupus erythematosus." Arth Rheum 16:4, 507-521, 1973.

41. Q. Discuss aseptic meningitis as a complication of systemic lupus erythematosus.

A. Aseptic meningitis is a relatively infrequent manifestation of systemic lupus erythematosus. Neck rigidity, increased CSF pressures, increased protein, and a mild lymphocytic pleocytosis are typically present. Of significance is the fact that aseptic meningitis may herald the development of more serious central nervous systemic involvement with lupus cerebritis.

REF: Canoso, J.J. and Cohen, A.S. "Aseptic meningitis in systemic lupus erythematosus." Arth Rheum 18:4, 369-374, 1975.

42. Q. What is the frequency of hypertension in systemic lupus erythematosus and discuss its relationship to renal failure?

A. Hypertension is felt to occur in approximately 45% of patients with systemic lupus erythematosus. It is frequently an early finding and not necessarily associated with renal failure. Approximately two thirds of hypertensive lupus patients had creatinine clearances of 60 cc min. or more.

REF: Budman, D.R. and Steinberg, A.D. "Hypertension and renal disease in systemic lupus erythematosus." Arch Intern Med 136, 1003-1007, 1976.

43. Q. Discuss the salient features of avascular necrosis in systemic lupus erythematosus.

A. Avascular necrosis of bone appears to have a predilection for young patients with systemic lupus erythematosus. A diagnosis of avascular necrosis should be considered when persistent localized joint pain develops. The clinical setting is frequently that of a lupus patient who is in a relative remission and who may in fact be relatively active with increased physical activity, during which time increased activity may precipitate articular collapse. Treatment with corticosteroid medication does not appear to be a major factor in the development of avascular necrosis.

REF: Smith, F.E., Sweet, D.E., Brunner, C.M., and Davis, J.S., IV. "Avascular necrosis in SLE." Ann Rheum Dis 35, 227-232, 1976.

44. Q. In studies of systemic lupus erythematosus in families, discuss the results of such studies in the context of genetic and environmental factors.

A. Disease expression is similar among cases of familial lupus as contrasted to lupus symptomatology in unrelated controls. These data have been interpreted to suggest a genetic influence. On the other hand, the mode and time of initiation of lupus appears to be governed, at least in part, by environmental factors. This is especially noteworthy in siblings.

REF: Arnett, F.C. and Shulman, L.E. "Studies in familial systemic lupus erythematosus." Medicine 55:4, 313-339, 1976.

45. Q. Discuss the relative yield of various neurological studies in the diagnosis of central nervous system involvement in systemic lupus erythematosus.

A. No single test or procedure is uniformly diagnostic in central nervous system involvement in systemic lupus erythematosus. However, the following battery of tests appears to be most useful: elevated CSF protein (38%), increased CSF-IgG (69%), decreased CSF hemolytic C4 (10%), increased CSF anti-DNA (64%), electroencephalogram abnormalities (80%), flow brain scan abnormalities (50%).

REF: Small, P., Mass M. F., Kohler, P. F., and Harbeck, R. J. "Central Nervous systemic involvement in SLE." Arth Rheum 20:3, 869-878, 1977.

46. Q. Discuss the "lupus anticoagulant" as to its nature and its clinical significance in terms of producing a bleeding diathesis.

A. Several coagulation defects have been described in systemic lupus erythematosus including circulating anticoagulants directed against factors XII, XI, IX, and VIII. However, the most common anti-coagulant is a complex that blocks the activation of prothrombin by prothrombin activator (Xa, V, and phospholipid). This results in a prolonged activated partial thromboplastin time (PTT) and a mildly prolonged prothrombin time (PT). In general, there appears to be little clinical significance in these patients with only one episode of excessive bleeding in 18 patients undergoing surgical procedures.

REF: Boxer, M., Ellman, L., and Carvalho, A. "The lupus anticoagulant." Arth Rheum 19:6, 1244-1248, 1976.

47. Q. What is the correlation between the lupus band-test and evidence of disease activity such as renal disease?

A. The lupus band-test refers to deposits of immunoglobulin and complement components at the dermal-epidermal junction in the skin of lupus patients. Such deposits occur in uninvolved skin in 40-60% of patients. However, there appears to be no significant clinical correlation with other parameters of activity in SLE, including nephritis, renal histology, hypocomplementemia, or the level of anti-DNA antibodies.

REF: Wertheimer, D. and Barland, P. "Clinical significance of immune deposits in the skin in SLE." Arth Rheum 19:6, 1249-1254, 1976.

48. Q. Discuss the various hematological abnormalities common to systemic lupus erythematosus.

A. Anemia is seen in perhaps 50% of patients with active systemic lupus erythematosus, and in the majority of these patients is associated with anemia of "chronic disease." Only 10% of patients with a Coomb's positive test manifest evidence of hemolysis. Autoantibodies may occur and lead to leukopenia affecting both the granulocytic and lymphocytic lines. Thrombocytopenia occurs usually as the result of increased peripheral destruction of platelets due to immune mechanisms. Qualitative abnormalities in platelet function may also occur as may various anti-coagulants, especially to the activation of prothrombin. However, despite these defects in platelets and coagulation factors, spontaneous bleeding is uncommon. Lymphocyte-typing techniques have revealed an over-activity of B-lymphocytes, perhaps due to a loss of regulatory T-cell function. Treatment with corticosteroid medication is generally therapeutically effective in most hematological problems, although splenectomy or treatment with immunosuppressive agents may be necessary.

REF: Budman, D.R. and Steinberg, A.D. "Hematologic aspects of systemic lupus erythematosus." <u>Ann Intern Med</u> 86:220-229, 1977.

49. Q. What is the correlation between levels of anti-DNA antibodies and evidence of clinical activity in systemic lupus erythematosus?

A. In nearly all cases of active systemic lupus erythematosus the anti-DNA titer is elevated. Of 206 sera tested only 4 had normal levels of this antibody. However, the anti-DNA antibody titer may remain elevated despite clinical remission, as evidenced by mild to moderate elevations in 34 sera at the time of clinical remission. Although the anti-DNA titer remains a useful parameter in SLE, decisions regarding therapy should not be based on this test alone.

REF: Davis, P., Percy, J.S., and Russell, A.S. "Correlation between levels of DNA antibodies and clinical disease activity in SLE." <u>Ann Rheum Dis</u> 36:157-159, 1977.

50. Q. What is the relative usefulness of the antinuclear
antibody test as compared to the anti-DNA titer in evalua-
ting disease activity in systemic lupus erythematosus and
what is the correlation between these two tests?

      A. Both the antinuclear antibody and the anti-DNA
titer are useful in the diagnosis of systemic lupus erythematosus, although homogeneous antinuclear antibody patterns are also commonly seen in SLE. However, in evaluation of disease activity, the anti-DNA titer shows greater
correlation between parameters of clinical activity than the
peripheral-staining antinuclear antibody titer. Anti-DNA
titers correlated well with severity of renal disease, decreased serum complement levels, and number of SLE
criteria. Peripheral-staining antinuclear antibody titers
did not show good correlation between disease activity or
the anti-DNA titer.

REF: Weitzman, R. J. and Walker, S. E. "Relation of
titred peripheral pattern ANA to anti-DNA and disease activity in systemic lupus erythematosus." Ann Rheum Dis
36:44-49, 1977.

51. Q. Discuss the typical course of membranous lupus
nephropathy.

      A. Unlike previous reports in the literature concern-
ing the clinical course of membranous glomerulonephritis
due to systemic lupus erythematosus, recent studies suggest that the course in this type of renal lesion is often
stable over many years. Proteinuria is usually persistent
despite treatment with corticosteroids. Only a minority of
patients demonstrate progressive renal disease, and generally this is a slowly deteriorating pattern. Therefore, it
may be concluded that membranous lupus nephritis is often
a benign disorder compatible with many years of stability in
renal function, as opposed to proliferative glomerulonephritis
in systemic lupus erythematosus.

REF: Donadio, J. V., Jr., Burgess, J. H., and Holley,
K. E. "Membranous lupus nephropathy: A clinico-pathologic
study." Medicine 56:6, 527-536, 1977.

52. Q. What is the significance of antibodies to cytoplasmic antigens in systemic lupus erythematosus?

A. Anticytoplasmic antibodies may represent a serological marker for systemic involvement in lupus erythematosus. In patients with cutaneous lupus, the presence of these antibodies suggests systemic disease. Furthermore, there appears to be a subpopulation of patients with clinical features resembling systemic lupus but without antinuclear antibodies. In this group of patients anticytoplasmic antibodies are frequently positive.

REF: Provost, T. T., Ahmed, A. R., Maddison, P. J., and Reichlin, M. "Antibodies to cytoplasmic antigens in lupus erythematosus." Arth Rheum 20.8, 1457-1463, 1977.

53. Q. Deficiencies of complement components have been described in association with which rheumatic disorders?

A. Systemic lupus erythematosus has been described in association with a number of complement component deficiencies. These include C2, C4, C5, and C8. Vasculitic syndromes have also been linked to deficiency of the second component of complement. Dermatomyositis has been found to be present in a patient with C2 deficiency, while Raynaud's phenomenon has been associated with C7.

REF: Schaller, J. G., Gilliland, B. G., Ochs, H. D., et. al "Severe systemic lupus erythematosus with nephritis in a boy with deficiency of the fourth component of complement." Arth Rheum 20:8, 1519-1524, 1977.

54. Q. Patients with systemic lupus erythematosus may have evidence of renal involvement by histological and immunofluorescent criteria without clinically apparent abnormalities. Please comment.

A. A wide range of abnormalities may be found histologically on renal biopsy in patients with systemic lupus erythematosus who have normal renal function by conventional laboratory parameters. These abnormalities include focal and proliferative glomerulonephritis, thickening of the basement membrane, and subendothelial deposits. Electronmicroscopy confirms the presence of mild to moderately severe abnormalities. Immunofluorescence demonstrates deposition of IgG, IgM, and complement. Therefore, it may be said that patients with systemic lupus erythematosus may have early evidence of renal involvement by histological and immunofluorescent criteria despite completely normal laboratory testing of renal function.

REF: Mahajan, S. K., Ordonez, N. G., Feitelson, P. J. et. al. "Lupus nephropathy without clinical renal involvement." Medicine 56:6, 493-501, 1977.
Hollcraft, R. M., Dubois, E. L., Lundberg, G. D., et. al. "Renal damage in systemic lupus erythematosus with normal renal function." J Rheum 3:3, 251-260, 1976.

55. Q. Characterize asymptomatic pulmonary involvement in systemic lupus erythematosus.

A. A study of patients with systemic lupus erythematosus who were free of pulmonary symptoms revealed restricted lung volumes and vital capacity. Although diffusing capacity was also reduced, the reduction was in proportion to the reduction in lung volumes. It has been hypothesized that these early changes noted in pulmonary function may be due to pulmonary thickening.

REF: Chick, T. W., DeHoratius, R. J., Skipper, B. E. and Messner, R. P. "Pulmonary dysfunction in systemic lupus erythematosus without pulmonary symptoms." J Rheum 3:3, 262-268, 1976.

56. Q. In family studies of systemic lupus erythematosus, what are the relative contributions of environmental factors as opposed to genetic factors in the pathogenesis of lupus erythematosus.

A. From a number of clinical studies, both environmental factors as well as genetic factors have emerged as being of some importance in the pathogenesis of systemic lupus erythematosus. C-type viruses have been implicated as environmental factors. Positive skin biopsies for deposits of immunofluorescent immunoglobulin and complement occur with greater frequency in household contacts of patients with lupus erythematosus irrespective of consanguinity. This finding also suggests the importance of environmental factors. On the other hand, serological data suggest that genetic factors are of significance. Anti-nuclear antibodies have been identified in higher titers in relatives of patients with lupus as compared to spouses. The occurance of lupus in twins further strengthens the role of genetic factors in this disease.

REF: Lowenstein, M.B., and Rothfield, N. F. "Family study of systemic lupus erythematosus." Arth Rheum 20:7, 1293-1303, 1977.

57. Q. Describe the hand deformities in systemic lupus erythematosus and comment on the type of surgical correction that is possible.

A. Subluxation and dislocation of the metacarpopha-langeal joints may be seen and can become irreducible. Swan neck deformities and Boutonniere deformities occur as well. These deformities are felt to be the result of contractures of the soft tissues. Erosive disease, in con-trast to rheumatoid deformities, is absent. The treatment of choice is to perform metacarpal osteotomy and shorten-ing in an attempt to decompress the contracted soft tissues. Joint replacement is not indicated in view of the usual preservation of articular cartilage.

REF: Evans, J.A., Hastings, D.E., and Urowitz, M.B. "The fixed lupus hand deformity and its surgical correction." J Rheum 4:2, 170-175, 1977.

58. Q. With the use of immunostimulants such as levami-sole in the treatment of rheumatoid arthritis, what is the clinical significance of positive antinuclear antibody titers in patients with rheumatoid arthritis?

A. There is clinical evidence that suggests a correla-tion between the phytohemagglutinin stimulation of lympho-cytes and antinuclear antibody titers in patients with rheu-matoid arthritis. In rheumatoid arthritic patients with positive antinuclear antibody titers, depressed lymphocyte responsiveness was noted. However, in rheumatoid pa-tients with negative antinuclear antibody titers, normal lymphocyte responsiveness was present. It has therefore been suggested that the antinuclear antibody test may serve as a useful marker in identifying that subpopulation of rheumatoid patients who could perhaps benefit from immunostimulant therapy.

REF: Menard, H.A., Dion, J., and Richard, C. "Antinuclear antibody: Predictive of lymphocyte response in rheumatoid arthritis." J Rheum 4:1, 21-26, 1977.

59. Q. Comment on the significance of C-reactive protein in systemic lupus erythematosus and contrast this to rheumatoid arthritis.

A. Rheumatoid arthritis is frequently characterized by a positive test for C-reactive protein. However, in systemic lupus erythematosus, C-reactive protein is generally absent. A notable exception is found in lupus patients with a superimposed infection of some type. During the period of active infection, the C-reactive protein becomes positive and later disappears from the convalescent sera of patients appropriately treated.

REF: Honig, S., Gorevic, P., and Weissmann, G. "C-reactive protein in systemic lupus erythematosus." Arth Rheum 20:5, 1065-1070, 1977.

60. Q. What is the significance of antibodies to nuclear ribonucleoprotein and Sm-antigen in systemic lupus erythematosus?

A. The Sm-antigen and its antibody have been closely correlated to systemic lupus erythematosus with a tendency toward more severe disease, nephritis, and positive anti-DNA titers. The antibody to ribonucleoprotein has been associated with the Mixed Connective Tissue syndrome by definition. However, perhaps 25% of lupus patients have positive titers of antibody to ribonucleoprotein. In these patients, the presence of antibody to ribonucleoprotein appears to be correlated with a benign prognosis, the absence of renal disease, and absent anti-DNA titers of high degree. It has therefore been suggested that a very important prognostic sign in patients with either a mixed connective tissue disorder or systemic lupus erythematosus is the absence or presence of antibody to ribonucleoprotein.

REF: Reichlin, M. "Problems in differentiating SLE and mixed connective tissue disease." N Engl J Med 295:21, 1194-1195, 1976.

61. Q. Discuss the lupus-like features of the NZB mouse and its hybrids in terms of the preliminary diagnostic criteria proposed for systemic lupus erythematosus.

A. The NZB mouse spontaneously develops certain features of systemic lupus erythematosus. Hemolytic anemia occurs in all mice, and glomerulonephritis in most (but not all). There are no LE cells, and therefore the NZB hybrid mouse, on the other hand, develops glomerulonephritis, positive LE cells and antinuclear antibodies, leukopenia and hemolytic anemia, thereby meeting four of the diagnostic criteria. Lymphoma is also known to develop in these mice in contrast to human lupus erythematosus.

REF: Wigley, R. D. "Models of rheumatic disease occuring spontaneously in mice." Sem Arth Rheum 7:2, 81-95, 1977.

62. Q. Compare and contrast the lupus-like syndrome seen in deficiency states of the second component of complement and systemic lupus erythematosus.

A. Patients with C2 deficiency differ from patients with SLE in having a greater frequency of disseminated discoid skin lesions, infrequent renal disease, low incidence of antibodies to native DNA, and a lack of granular immunoglobulin or complement deposition in the dermal-epidermal junction on skin biopsy.

REF: Agnello, V. "Complement deficiency states." Medicine 57:1, 1-23, 1977.

63. Q. Catalogue the clinical manifestations of systemic lupus erythematosus per organ system.

A. Systemic lupus erythematosus is truly a multisystemic disorder. Seven major organ systems may be involved. (1) Skin involvement includes the classical "butterfly" rash, diffuse skin lesions which may simulate dermatomyositis, discoid lupus lesions, oral ulcerations, and alopecia. (2) Articular involvement includes monoarticular or polyarticular synovitis which is usually nonerosive and nondeforming. (3) Renal disease may be seen from benign glomerulitis to life endangering glomerulonephritis. (4) Serous membranes may be inflamed, producing pleurisy, pericarditis, or peritonitis. (5) Hematological problems include leukopenia, hemolytic anemia, and thrombocytopenia. (6) Nervous system disorders range from seizures and psychosis, to peripheral neuritis and mononeuritis multiplex. (7) Pulmonary disease includes interstitial fibrosis and other progressive manifestations.

REF: Fries, J. F. "The clinical aspects of systemic lupus erythematosus." In Med Clin North Am, 61:2, 229-240, 1977.

64. Q. Discuss the clinical features of "canine lupus" as a model for the human counterpart of systemic lupus erythematosus.

A. "Canine lupus" first described in 1965 has become an important model for human lupus erythematosus. Common features of "canine lupus" include the following: hemolytic anemia, thrombocytopenia, leukopenia, polyarthritis, glomerulonephritis, "butterfly" rash, alopecia, pleuropericarditis, myositis, hepatomegaly, splenomegaly, lymphadenopathy, and lymphocytic thyroiditis.

REF: Steinberg, A. D. and Reinertsen, J. L. "Lupus in New Zealand Mice and Dogs." Bull Rheum Dis 28:4, 5, 940-947, 1977-78.

65. Q. How does "canine lupus" differ from human lupus erythematosus serologically?

A. "Canine lupus" is primarily a hematological disease. Although positive lupus cell preparations are commonly found, antibodies to native DNA are far less frequently a feature than is the case in human lupus. In "canine lupus" antibodies to single stranded DNA and RNA are more frequently noted, on the other hand, than in human lupus.

REF: Steinberg, A.D., and Reinertsen, J.L. "Lupus in New Zealand Mice and Dogs." Bull Rheum Dis 28:4, 5, 940-947, 1977-78.

66. Q. Using the models of lupus in mice and in dogs, discuss the current concepts of pathogenesis of systemic lupus erythematosus in human beings.

A. Systemic lupus erythematosus is a multifactorial disorder. Genetic factors have been implicated in the research with NZB mice, while environmental factors have been given considerable attention in studies with dogs and "canine lupus." It would appear that multiple factors are involved, including genetic, viral, biochemical and hormonal factors. Variable effects on the immune system and such parameters as B-cell stimulation, T-cell suppression, and the immunobiological role of immune complexes are all relevant factors in the pathogenesis of this disorder.

REF: Steinberg, A.D., and Reinertsen, J.L. "Lupus in New Zealand Mice and Dogs." Bull Rheum Dis 28:4, 5, 940-947, 1977-78.

III. SCLERODERMA

67. Q. Discuss the HLA tissue typing data in patients with classical progressive systemic sclerosis and the CREST syndrome.

A. There appears to be no significant preponderance of any of the HLA antigens in either progressive systemic sclerosis or in the CREST syndrome.

REF: Birnbaum, N.S., Rodnan, G.P., Rabin, B.S. and Bassion, S. "Histocompatibility antigens in progressive systemic sclerosis (scleroderma)." J Rheum 4:4, 425-428, 1978.

68. Q. Discuss the possibility of genetic factors in scleroderma from currently available data.

A. From familial studies several interesting facts have emerged. The frequency of serum antinuclear antibodies is increased in first degree relatives of patients with scleroderma and may be detected in 58% of cases. In addition, in some studies there have been chromosomal abnormalities noted in family members who have developed scleroderma. Familial scleroderma is being reported with greater frequency as well. As with other rheumatic diseases, it is hypothesized that genetic predisposition is of importance in scleroderma when combined with the proper and as yet unknown environmental stimulus.

REF: Gray, R.G. and Altman, R.D. "Progressive systemic sclerosis in a family." Arth Rheum 20:1, 35-40, 1977.

69. Q. Describe the esophageal abnormalities in scleroderma.

A. Diminished or absent contractility of the esophagus may occur in scleroderma and in the CREST syndrome, and appears to be correlated with Raynaud's phenomenon. The lower third of the esophagus is most frequently involved.

Severe dysphagia and acid reflux may lead to stricture and esophageal ulceration.

REF: Ramirez Mata, M., Ibanex, G., and Alarcon Segovia, D. "Stimulatory effect of metoclopramide on the esophagus and lower esophageal sphincter of patients with PSS." Arth Rheum 20:1, 30-34, 1977.

70. Q. In preliminary studies, what mode of treatment appears promising in patients with scleroderma who develop severe esophageal motility disturbances, which heretofore have been untreatable?

A. A smooth muscle stimulant, metoclopramide is a procainamide derivative with effects on the medullary region as well as direct effects on the esophageal and gastrointestinal tract. In preliminary studies, it appears that this drug may improve the symptoms of esophageal motility disturbances in PSS by increasing the sphincteric pressure and generating esophageal contractility.

REF: McCallum, R.W., Ippoliti, A.F., Cooney, C., and Sturdevant, R.A.L. "A controlled trial of metoclopramide in symptomatic gastroesophageal reflux." New Engl J Med 296:7, 354-357, 1977.

71. Q. What is the characteristic histological pattern in the blood vessels affected by scleroderma?

A. Small and medium sized arteries and arterioles are typically involved. Intimal proliferation with narrowing of the lumen appears to be the most significant alteration, although changes in the media also may be found. This pattern is duplicated in the digital vessels in Raynaud's phenomenon, the lung in pulmonary hypertension, and the kidney in sclerodermatous renal involvement.

REF: Salerni, R., Rodnan, G.P., Leon, D.F., and Shaver, J.A. "Pulmonary hypertension in the CREST syndrome variant of progressive systemic sclerosis (scleroderma)." Ann Intern Med 86, 394-399, 1977.

72. Q. Describe what is meant by the CREST syndrome
and comment on this form of scleroderma as a benign
variant.

A. The CREST syndrome refers to a variant of scleroderma with the elements of calcinosis, Raynaud's phenomenon, esophageal motility abnormalities, sclerodactyly,
and telangiectasias. It has long been considered a benign
form of scleroderma. Some patients, however, may progress to the development of typical progressive systemic
sclerosis after many years of observation, while other patients may develop widespread intestinal abnormalities,
pulmonary hypertension, and cor pulmonale.

REF: Salerni, R. , Rodnan, G. P. , Leon, D. F. , and Shaver,
J. A. "Pulmonary hypertension in the CREST syndrome
variant of progressive systemic sclerosis (scleroderma). "
Ann Intern Med 86, 394-399, 1977.

73. Q. Comment on the immunoglobulin and complement
system in the vascular lesions of scleroderma as found in
the kidney or in the pulmonary vasculature.

A. The role of immunoglobulins and complement is
far from settled in scleroderma. However, some studies
have localized IgG and certain complement components to
the interlobular renal arteries and the pulmonary arterioles
in scleroderma. Their significance is unknown at this time.

REF: Gerber, M. A. "Immunohistochemical findings in the
renal vascular lesions of progressive systemic sclerosis."
Hum Pathol 6, 343-347, 1975.

74. Q. Describe the various forms of scleroderma in
childhood.

A. The most common form of sclerodermatous involvement in childhood is that of local lesions of various
kinds which may be multiple. Interference with growth,
joint, soft tissue, and tendon contractures may produce progressive deformities. Diffuse and systemic forms of scleroderma may also occur, but are seen far less frequently than

the localized forms. A rare third variant has been referred to as sclerodermatous fasciitis.

REF: Ansell, B.M., Nasseh, G.A., and Bywaters, E.G.L. "Scleroderma in childhood." Ann Rheum Dis 35, 190-197, 1976.

75. Q. Discuss the serological manifestations of sclero-derma as seen in children.

A. In general, the antinuclear antibody is positive and there may be a generalized gammaglobulinemia. However, tests for rheumatoid factor are negative, there does not appear to be a significant anti-DNA binding titer, and complement levels remain relatively normal.

REF: Answell, B.M., Nasseh, G.A., and Bywaters, E.G.L. "Scleroderma in childhood." Ann Rheum Dis 35, 190-197, 1976.

76. Q. Discuss the patterns of finger capillary abnormalities seen in scleroderma and other connective tissue disorders.

A. In scleroderma, the typical pattern is that of mas-sive capillary dilatation, which may also be noted in pa-tients with dermatomyositis. In rheumatoid arthritis, there appears to be a more prominent subpapillary plexus of the nailfold. In systemic lupus erythematosus, the pattern is that of focal deletion of capillaries with "punched out" lesions.

REF: Maricq, H.R. and LeRoy, C. "Patterns of finger capillary abnormalities in connective tissue diseases by "wide field" microscopy." Arth Rheum 15:5, 619-628, 1973.

77. Q. Discuss the feasibility of renal transplantation in patients with chronic renal failure from sclerodermatous kidney disease.

A. Several studies have now appeared that suggest successful transplantation of compatible donor kidneys may be accomplished without return of scleroderma in the donor kidney. However, there are also reports that suggest a recurrence. Further data will be important, but at this time the possibility of renal transplatation would be feasible in an otherwise reasonably healthy patient with progressive renal failure from scleroderma kidney disease.

REF: Keane, W. F., Danielson, B., and Raij, L. "Successful renal transplatation in progressive systemic sclerosis." Ann Intern Med 85, 199-202, 1976.

Woodhall, P.B., McCoy, R.C., Gunnells, J.C. and Seigler, H. F. "Apparent recurrence of progressive systemic sclerosis in a renal allograft." JAMA 236:9, 1032- 1976.

78. Q. What are the most frequent presenting signs and symptoms in scleroderma?

A. Sclerodermatous skin changes are the most commonly seen abnormality and occur in 90 to 98% of cases. Raynaud's phenomenon is seen in approximately 80%, and abnormalities of esophageal function in 50 to 75%.

REF: Siegel, R.C. "Scleroderma." In Med Clin North Am 61:2, 283-297, 1977.

79. Q. Describe the types of internal organ involvement seen in progressive systemic sclerosis and estimate their frequency of occurrence as clinical entities.

A. Pulmonary involvement (43%) and cardiac disease (40%) appear to be the most frequently seen manifestations. Kidney disorders occur in about one third of patients. Musculoskeletal manifestations account for 20 to 25%. Pericarditis and intestinal involvement are present in 10 to 15% of patients.

REF: Siegel, R.C. "Scleroderma." In Med Clin North Am 61:2, 283-297, 1977.

80. Q. Compare the frequency of internal organ involvement as it occurs in the clinical situation to evidence of such involvement at autopsy.

A. When autopsy statistics are compared to clinical incidence, it becomes apparent that internal organ involvement of the heart, lungs, kidneys, intestinal tract, and esophagus occurs far more frequently than is generally clinically recognized. Sclerodermatous involvement of the esophagus occurs in 74% of cases, intestinal involvement in 46%, renal disease in 58%, and cardiopulmonary disease in 81%.

REF: Siegel, R.C. "Scleroderma." In Med Clin North Am 61:2, 283-297, 1977.

81. Q. Discuss the present status of treatment in sclero-derma.

A. Clearly, no satisfactory mode of treatment is known for scleroderma. The only exception to this rule is that of eosinophilic fasciitis or sclerodermatous fasciitis wherein treatment with corticosteroid medication appears to be high-ly beneficial. However, in the CREST syndrome or in pro-gressive systemic sclerosis, there is not convincing evi-dence for a reliable form of treatment. Corticosteroids are of little value, and some have suggested that they per-haps accelerate the development of renal disease. Initially, colchicine was reported in a favorable context, but more recent studies have failed to confirm a therapeutic role for skin manifestations. Penicillamine has had its proponents as has leukeran and other immunosuppressive drugs, but the data remains conflicting. Dimethylsulfoxide (DMSO) ap-pears promising in certain studies, although as yet no firm conclusions can be drawn.

REF: Siegel, R.C. "Scleroderma." In Med Clin North Am 61:2, 283-297, 1977.

82. Q. Comment on the frequency of association between Sjogren's syndrome and progressive systemic sclerosis.

A. Although early studies suggested a rather low inci-dence of Sjogren's syndrome in scleroderma, more recent studies attest to the fact that there is indeed a significant correlation between the occurance of these two disorders. Figures have ranged from a low of 0 to 5% and a high of greater than 90%. More recent figures suggest a prevalence figure of 17%.

REF: Cipoletti, J. F. , Buckingham, R. B. , Barnes, E. L. , et. al. "Sjogren's syndrome in progressive systemic sclerosis." <u>Ann Intern Med</u> 87, 535-541, 1977.

83. Q. What abnormalities of pulmonary function are common in scleroderma, and which of these would probably be the first to become abnormal?

A. Decreased diffusing capacity was most often seen in patients with restrictive disease, and rarely was it the only abnormality in pulmonary function. Restrictive disease and obstructive disease were noted in nearly 30% of patients, but small airway disease was present in over 40%. It was concluded by the authors that small airway disease was the most commonly seen pulmonary function abnormality and was perhaps the earliest to develop.

REF: Guttadauria, M. , Ellman, H. , Emmanuel, G. , et. al. "Pulmonary function in scleroderma." <u>Arth Rheum</u> 20:5, 1071-1078, 1977.

IV. POLYMYOSITIS AND DERMATOMYOSITIS
AND RELATED DISORDERS OF MUSCLE

84. Q. Describe the most useful diagnostic criteria for polymyositis and dermatomyositis.

A. The following criteria help to best define the spectrum of polymyositis and dermatomyositis: (1) Proximal and symmetrical muscular weakness, with or without dysphagia or respiratory muscle weakness; (2) the electromyographic triad characteristic of polymyositis; (3) typical muscle biopsy changes which include the presence of interstitial inflammatory cells; (4) elevation of the muscle enzymes in serum, including the CPK, aldolase, SGOT and SGPT, and the LDH. (5) When present, the dermatologic manifestations of dermatomyositis.

REF: Bohan, A. , Peter, J.B. , Bowman, R.L. , and Pearson, C.M. "A Computer-assisted analysis of 153 patients with polymyositis and dermatomyositis." Medicine 56:4, 255-286, 1977.

85. Q. What are the features of the typical "triad" as seen in the electromyogram of polymyositis and dermatomyositis?

A. The EMG "triad" seen in polymyositis and dermatomyositis consists of: (1) Short-duration, small-amplitude "myopathic" action potentials; (2) Increased membrane irritability which includes increased insertional irritability, spontaneous fibrillations, and positive sharp waves; and (3) abrupt, bizarre, high frequency bursts that have been termed "pseudomyotonic" discharges.

REF: Lambert, E.H. , Sayre, G.P. , and Eaton, L.M. Electrical activity of muscle in polymyositis. Trans Am Neurol Assoc 79:64-69, 1954.

86. Q. Discuss the concept of polymyositis and dermatomyositis in association with malignant disease.

A. Varying figures have been given in the literature concerning the frequency with which malignancy is seen in association with polymyositis, and more particularly with dermatomyositis. Figures as high as 71% have been quoted by Shy in men over the age of 50 years. Other figures have ranged from 15-34%. However, although the true frequency of this association is not known, most authorities believe that malignant disease occurs in about 10% of patients with polymyositis and dermatomyositis.

REF: Bohan, A., and Peter, J.B. N Engl J Med 292:344-347, and 403-407, 1975.

87. Q. What are the indications for the use of immuno-suppressive agents in polymyositis and dermatomyositis and which of these drugs have been found to be of most value?

A. Immunosuppressive drugs are still to be considered experimental in the treatment of polymyositis and dermatomyositis. In general, there are two main criteria for their use. Firstly, in a patient who has received the equivalent of prednisone, 40 mgm daily for at least 3 months, and who has not responded clinically with improvement in muscle strength, these drugs are then added for what is termed "steroid unresponsiveness." Secondly, in patients who have responded to corticosteroid medication, but who continue to require an unacceptably high steroid maintenance level, immunosuppressive medication is then added for "steroid sparing." Methotrexate has been the agent of choice, although various other immunosuppressive medications have been employed. These include azathioprine, cyclophosphamide, and leukeran.

REF: Metzger, A.L., Bohan, A., Goldberg, L.S., et.al. Ann Intern Med 81:182-189, 1974.

88. Q. Discuss the current concepts of the etiology and pathogenesis of polymyositis and dermatomyositis.

A. The cause of these disorders is not known. However, it has long been suspected that an immunological etiology is probable. The role of antibodies has been questioned because such antibodies to muscle are not cytotoxic and may be found in other disorders of muscle such as muscular dystrophy and neurogenic diseases. However, the demonstration of antigen-antibody complexes with complement by immunofluorescent techniques has raised the issue

of immunologically induced vasculitis as a possible pathogenetic mechanism. Perhaps the most convincing data may
be found in the area of delayed hypersensitivity where cytotoxicity has been demonstrated with lymphocytes as well as
lymphokines from patients with active polymyositis. The
role of viruses remain enigmatic. Some investigators believe that electron-microscopy has demonstrated viral-like
particles in muscle tissue from patients with polymyositis;
whereas others claim these are artefactual.

REF: Bohan, A., and Peter, J. B. "Polymyositis and
dermatomyositis." N Engl J Med 292:344-347, and 403-
407, 1975.

89. Q. What is the incidence of myoglobinemia in polymyositis?

A. Radioimmunoassay for serum myoglobin in patients
with polymyositis revealed elevated levels in 50% of patients. It has been suggested that the serum myoglobin level is perhaps a more sensitive indicator of disease activity.
Its use with the usual muscle enzymes has been advocated
in following the course of patients with polymyositis.

REF: Nishikai, M., and Reichlin, M. "Radioimmunoassay
of serum myoglobin in polymyositis and other conditions."
Arth and Rheum 20:8, 1514-1518, 1977.

90. Q. Describe the vascular abnormalities seen in polymyositis and dermatomyositis and comment on their
implications as to pathogenesis.

A. In polymyositis the following are most commonly
seen: endothelial swelling and degenerative changes, peri-
vascular mononuclear infiltrates, localization of IgG in intramuscular blood vessels, microtubular inclusions in endothelial cells, thickening of the basement membrane and
lamination. In dermatomyositis similar changes are also
found. Additionally, fibrin thrombus formation has been
described as well as fibrinoid necrosis of vessel walls, and
abnormalities in nailfold capillary patterns. It has been

suggested that such abnormalities may lead to muscle ischemia thereby resulting in some of the clinical manifestations seen in these disorders.

REF: Scherer, A. T., and Masi, A. T. "Polymyositis and other myopathy staining patterns with the new hematoxylin basic fuchsin picric acid (HBFP) method." J Rheum 3:3, 215-222, 1976.

91. Q. List the causes of rhabdomyolysis.

A. The causes of rhabdomyolysis have been classified as follows: (1) Increased energy consumption: exercise, heat stroke, malignant hyperthermia, fever, convulsions, delirium tremens, tetanus, amphetamines. (2) Decreased energy production due to genetic factors: phosphorylase deficiency, diabetic acidosis, hyperosmolar coma, carnitine deficiency. (3) Acquired defects leading to decreased energy production: hypokalemia, ethanol abuse, myxedema, hypothermia, hypophosphatemia. (4) Ischemic conditions of muscle: hypokalemia, crush syndrome, embolism. (5) Muscle injury: polymyositis and dermatomyositis, trauma, crush, burns. (6) Infections: gas gangrene, tetanus, leptospirosis, viral syndromes, coxsackie, shigellosis. (7) Miscellaneous causes such as venoms, drugs and ethylene glycol.

REF: Humphreys, M. H. "Rhabdomyolysis." West J Med 125:298-304, 1976.

92. Q. Discuss the typical laboratory findings in myoglobinuric acute renal failure.

A. The urine hematest is positive but there are no red blood cells in the sediment. The urine is positive for myoglobin. Hyperkalemia, hyperuricemia, hyperphosphatemia out of proportion to the degree of renal failure, and hypocalcemia early in the course are typical features. Later, hypercalcemia ensues. The BUN to creatinine ratio is less than 10:1. The muscle enzymes are elevated in the serum.

REF: Humphreys, M. H. "Rhabdomyolysis." West J Med 125:298-304, 1976.

93. Q. Discuss the factors that seem to influence survival in polymyositis and dermatomyositis.

A. There are no demographic, clinical, or laboratory features that predict survival characteristics in patients with polymyositis and dermatomyositis. The presence of an associated malignancy clearly lessens the survival, and because this is associated with increased age, then the latter becomes indirectly correlated with poor survival. Additionally, the presence of dysphagia or severe muscle weakness lessens the chances of survival.

REF: Carpenter, J.R., Bunch, T.W., Engel, A.G., and O'Brien, P.C. "Survival in polymyositis: Corticosteroids and risk factors." J Rheum 4:2, 207-214, 1977.

Bohan A., Peter, J.B., Bowman, R.L., et.al. "A computer assisted analysis of 153 patients with polymyositis and dermatomyositis." Medicine 56:4, 255-286, 1977.

94. Q. In a patient with hypertrophic cardiomyopathy, comment on the possibility of involvement of voluntary muscle.

A. In a study of patients with hypertrophic cardiomyopathy, electromyography and muscle biopsy suggested evidence of a mild myopathic disorder, which was minimally symptomatic on a clinical level. The authors suggested that this type of cardiomyopathy might represent a widespread process not necessarily completely restricted to the heart.

REF: Smith, E.R., Heffernan, L.P., Sangalang, V.E., et.al. "Voluntary muscle involvement in hypertrophic cardiomyopathy." Ann Intern Med 85:566-572, 1976.

95. Q. Discuss the periodic paralyses.

A. The periodic paralyses have been divided into primary and secondary types. The primary periodic paralyses in turn have been categorized into (a) Hypokalemic, (b) hyperkalemic, and (c) normokalemic varieties on the basis of the serum potassium during acute attacks. In addition, there is a fourth type, (e) paramyotonia congenita, which involves the induction of massive myotonia and weakness upon exposure to cold. Of the secondary types of periodic paralyses, endocrine dysfunction (thyrotoxicosis, aldosteronism), disorders of potassium (renal tubular acidosis, diabetic acidosis), and ingestion of large amounts of licorice may result in periodic paralysis.

REF: Pearson, C.M. and Kalyanaraman, K. "The periodic paralyses," in The Metabolic Basis of Inherited Disease, Third Edition, Ed. J.B. Stanbury, J.B. Wyngaarden, and D.S. Frederickson. McGraw Hill, Inc., 1972, p. 1181-1203.

96. Q. Describe the distinguishing clinical features of the hypokalemic type of periodic paralysis.

A. The onset is usually from 7 to 21 years of age, and the duration of attacks is on the order of several hours. Complete paralysis is frequent, although the facial muscles and respiratory muscles are spared. Patients often awaken paralyzed. The serum potassium is generally low during an attack.

REF: Pearson, C.M. and Kalyanaraman, K. "The periodic paralyses," in The Metabolic Basis of Inherited Disease, Third Edition, Ed. J.B. Stanbury, J.B. Wyngaarden, and D.S. Frederickson, McGraw Hill, Inc., 1972, p. 1181-1203.

97. Q. What are the clinical features of hyperkalemic periodic paralysis?

A. The onset is generally in the first decade of life with attacks lasting less than an hour or so. Weakness is typically relatively mild and may be localized. The serum potassium is typically elevated during an acute attack.

REF: Pearson, C.M. and Kalyanaraman, K. "The periodic paralyses," in The Metabolic Basis of Inherited Disease, Third Edition, Ed. J.B. Stanbury, J.B. Wyngaarden, and D.S. Frederickson, McGraw Hill, Inc., 1972, p. 1181-1203.

98. Q. Normokalemic periodic paralysis is the third
type of periodic paralysis. What are its clinical features?

A. The age of onset is in the first decade, and symptoms generally last from 2 days to 3 weeks. The paralysis
is severe and includes the jaw and cough reflexes. Patients
usually awaken paralyzed. The serum potassium is often
normal, although slight depression may be noted.

REF: Pearson, C.M. and Kalyanaraman, K. "The periodic
paralyses," In The Metabolic Basis of Inherited Disease,
Third Edition, Ed. J.B. Stanbury, J.B. Wyngaarden, and
D.S. Frederickson, McGraw Hill, Inc., 1972, p. 1181-
1203.

99. Q. Describe the effect on muscle enzymes in serum
of exercise in patients with motor neuron disease and
weakness of muscle.

A. When patients with motor neuron disorders and muscular atrophy are subjected to exercise, there is an elevation
of the serum enzymes, most notably the CPK, which parallels
a similar rise seen in normal controls who have also exercised.
However, in general, the serum levels of CPK in the resting
state are normal in controls, whereas they are elevated in patients with motor neuron muscular atrophy. The implications
of these observations are that in a patient with motor neuron
disease who is at rest, the CPK level represents that which is
at near maximal efflux from necrotic muscle cells, and that any
further increase in the CPK comes from exercise induced efflux from relatively normal muscle fibers.

REF: Welch, K.M. and Goldberg, D.M. "Response of serum enzymes and other biochemical constituents to strenu-
ous exercise in control subjects and patients with motor
neuron disease." J Neurol Sci 19, 225-234, 1973.

100. Q. Describe the muscle enzyme pattern which may be
seen in motor neuron disorders, spinal muscular atrophy,
and amyotrophic lateral sclerosis.

A. Muscle enzymes have been noted to be elevated in
polymyositis and dermatomyositis. These enzymes may also be elevated in certain types of muscular dystrophy. However, it has not generally been appreciated that muscle

enzyme elevation in serum may be seen in a variety of neurogenic disorders, including motor neuron diseases such as the Kugelberg-Welander syndrome, and amyotrophic lateral sclerosis. The degree of muscle enzyme elevation may be slight, but may also be excessive, and as high as fourfold.

REF: Panitch, H. S., and Franklin, G. M. "Elevation of serum phosphokinase in amyotrophic lateral sclerosis." Neurology, 22:9, 964-966, 1972.

101. Q. Describe myositis fibrosa generalisata, and compare this to Stiff-Man Syndrome.

A. This is a very rare muscular disorder in which the muscles become rigid and firm, being replaced by fibrous tissue. Similarities to the stiff-man syndrome may occur, although there are also important differences. In general, the muscle biopsy in the stiff-man syndrome is relatively normal, while in myositis fibrosa the muscle fibers are replaced by sheets of fibrous tissue. Muscle enzymes may be elevated in the latter, while they are typically normal in the stiff-man syndrome. Finally, the stiff-man syndrome responds clinically to diazepam and is generally a nonprogressive disorder, whereas myositis fibrosa does not respond to diazepam and may be a fatal disease.

REF: Seitz, K. R. and Trostdorf, E. "Myositis fibrosa generalisata and Stiff-Man syndrome." Europ Neurol 3, 13-27, 1970.

102. Q. In an army platoon undergoing basic training, what effect on serum muscle enzymes would you expect to see and what would be the frequency of significant myoglobinemia?

A. In a study of over 300 recruits, a striking 39% had significantly elevated serum myoglobin levels. Many of these were completely asymptomatic. Serum muscle enzyme elevation was often striking, with CPK values as high as 10,000 mU per ml.

REF: Olerud, J. E., Homer, L. D., and Carroll, H. W. "Incidence of acute exertional rhabdomyolysis." Arch Intern Med 136, 692-697, 1976.

103. Q. Discuss the acute renal failure of rhabdomyolysis due to drug abuse or ethanol intoxication.

A. Lethargy or coma is generally associated with markedly elevated serum enzymes, especially the CPK and aldolase. Myoglobinemia, hyperuricemia, hyperkalemia, and a disproportionately increased serum creatinine concentration in relation to the serum BUN are characteristic features. Transient hypercalcemia may develop during the diuretic phase. The overall prognosis is relatively favorable, however, despite the severe catabolism.

REF: Koffler, A., Friedler, R.M., and Massry, S.G. "Acute renal failure due to nontraumatic rhabdomyolysis," Ann Intern Med 85, 23-28, 1976.

104. Q. Discuss the significance of the acetylcholine receptor antibody in myasthenia gravis.

A. In perhaps 70 percent of patients with myasthenia gravis, antibodies to acetylcholine receptor sites may be demonstrated. More than one receptor factor is present. The precise role of these antibodies has not yet been completely defined, although they serve to identify the disease and suggest further research efforts.

REF: Appel, S.H., Almon R.R., and Levy, N. "Acetylcholine receptor antibodies in myasthenia gravis." New Eng J Med 293:15, 760-761, 1975.

105. Q. In patients with inflammatory myopathies such as polymyositis, dermatomyositis, scleroderma, and so forth, what is the frequency of myoglobinemia, whether symptomatic or not?

A. In 74% of sera collected from patients with various forms of inflammatory myopathy, significant levels of serum myoglobin were detected. The level of myoglobinemia tended to correlate with serum enzymes and clinical weakness. In general, levels of myoglobinemia fell to normal before the muscle enzymes and provided a relatively good indication of disease activity.

REF: Kagen, L. J. "Myoglobinemia in inflammatory myopathies." JAMA 237:14, 1448-1452, 1977.

V. THE VASCULITIDES

106. Q. In patients with Hepatitis B infections, what are
the typical features that may be seen in terms of rheumatic
complaints?

A. Patients with Hepatitis B infections, whether they
become jaundiced or not, may present with basically one of
two ways with rheumatologic symptoms. Firstly, a systemic polyarthritic syndrome may be seen involving multiple joints, which may resemble rheumatoid arthritis. Secondly, a diffuse vasculitic syndrome may appear resembling
that which might be seen as part of the polyarteritis
spectrum.

REF: Duffy, J., Lidsky, M.D., Sharp, J.T., et.al. "Polyarthritis, polyarteritis and hepatitis B." Medicine 55:1, 19-
37, 1976.

107. Q. Describe the rheumatic complaints seen in hepatitis B infections presenting with primarily polyarthritic
symptoms.

A. These patients are typically quite ill with fever
and often a diffuse skin rash. Polyarticular arthritis is the
rule. In some cases, the rheumatoid factor may be positive,
even strongly so. The antinuclear antibody titer is generally negative, although low levels of antinuclear antibody
have been noted in a few patients. The serum complement
may be reduced, but may also remain in the normal range.
Therapeutic response to salicylates in the majority of patients
is prompt.

REF: Duffy, J., Lidsky, M.D., Sharp, J.T., et.al. "Polyarthritis, polyarteritis and hepatitis B." Medicine 55:1, 19-
37, 1976.

108. Q. In patients with hepatitis B infections, describe
the vasculitis that has been described.

A. A syndrome that resembles polyarteritis nodosa
has been associated with hepatitis B infections. The onset
may be either abrupt and life threatening, or may be a

relatively insidious one with progressive chronic debility.
Evidence of necrotizing vasculitis and glomerulonephritis
may be present. High fever, anemia, leukocytosis, multisystemic organ involvement, central nervous system involvement, gastrointestinal infarction, and cardiac involvement may appear and a fatal outcome may ensue.

REF: Duffy, J., Lidsky, M.D., Sharp, J.T., et.al. "Polyarthritis, polyarteritis and hepatitis B." Medicine 55:1, 19-
37, 1976.

109. Q. In patients who present with either the polyarthritic or vasculitic forms of rheumatic involvement, discuss
the presence of hepatitis-B antigen, hepatitis-B antibody,
and liver function test abnormalities in these patients.

A. It is important to recognize that patients with hepatitis-B infections may present with symptoms which are
principally rheumatological in nature. Jaundice may be absent throughout the entire course of the illness. Symptoms
may mimic those that might occur in classical polyarteritis
or rheumatoid arthritis. Additionally, the rheumatoid factor may be positive in the blood and may cause diagnostic
confusion. However, the liver function tests are almost invariably abnormal, and the serologic tests for hepatitis-B
antigen and hepatitis-B antibody are universally positive.

REF: Duffy, J., Lidsky, M.D., Sharp, J.T., et.al. "Polyarthritis, polyarteritis and hepatitis-B." Medicine 55:1, 19-
37, 1976.

110. Q. What percentage of patients with diffuse, chronic
vasculitis appear to have positive serological tests of hepatitis-B antigen? What significance does the vasculitis seen
with hepatitis-B have in terms of pathogenetic mechanisms?

A. It has been estimated that perhaps 30% of patients
with vasculitis have the hepatitis-B antigen in their blood.
This relationship represents evidence for the first instance
of a viral infection as a cause of chronic rheumatic disease
in man.

REF: Sergent, J.S., Lockshin, M.D., Christian, C.L.,
and Gocke, D.J. "Vasculitis with hepatitis-B antigenemia."
Medicine 55:1, 1-18, 1976.

111. Q. Discuss the differences in clinical presentation between hepatitis-B positive and negative patients with vasculitis.

A. There is no significant difference in the symptoms or modes of presentation between hepatitis-B positive and negative patients with the syndrome of diffuse, chronic vasculitis. In both groups, there appears to be no correlation between the vasculitic disease and the intensity of the liver involvement. Liver function tests are abnormal to an equal extent in both groups.

REF: Sergent, J.S., Lockshin, M.D., Christian, C.L., and Gocke, D.J. "Vasculitis with hepatitis-B antigenemia." Medicine 55:1, 1-18, 1976.

112. Q. Discuss the desirability and feasibility of alternate-day corticosteroids in the management of giant cell arteritis.

A. It is now well known that the use of corticosteroid medication in an alternate-day schedule reduces the complications of corticosteroids. However, despite the desirability of using an alternate-day regimen, it would appear that giant cell arteritis cannot be suppressed adequately with these agents unless corticosteroid drugs are administered on a daily basis.

REF: Hunder, G.G., Sheps, S.G., Allen G.L., and Joyce, J.W. "Daily and alternate-day corticosteroid regimens in treatment of giant cell arteritis." Ann Intern Med 82, 613-618, 1975.

113. Q. Describe the classical pathological signs of polyarteritis nodosa.

A. Medium sized arteries are typically affected in polyarteritis. The pathological hallmarks are swelling and fibrinoid necrosis of the media, polymorphonuclear cell infiltration of the wall of the blood vessel, chronic granulation tissue invasion with segmental weakening and aneurysmal dilatation, and obliteration of the lumen by fibrosis and scar formation.

REF: Boyle, J.A. and Buchanan, W.W. "Clinical Rheumatology." Blackwell Scientific Publications, Oxford and Edinburgh, 1971, 522.

114. Q. Polyarteritis nodosa may present with a multiplicity of syndromes, although in general three classical modes of presentation have been described by some authors. Discuss these.

A. (1) Hypertension, usually of relatively abrupt onset, with a rapidly accelerating course.
(2) Glomerulonephritis with proteinuria, casts, and diminishing renal function.
(3) Symmetrical peripheral neuritis or mononeuritis multiplex lesions.

REF: Boyle, J.A. and Buchanan, W.W. "Clinical Rheumatology." Blackwell Scientific Publications, Oxford and Edinburgh, 1971, p. 552.

115. Q. Describe Cogan's syndrome.

A. This is considered a variant of polyarteritis in which there is the combination of interstitial keratitis of non-syphilitic origin together with deafness. The syndrome is generally found in young adults.

REF: Boyle, J.A. and Buchanan, W.W. "Clinical Rheumatology." Blackwell Scientific Publications, Oxford and Edinburgh, 1971, p. 526.

116. Q. What kinds of evidence, both clinical and laboratory, would suggest that polyarteritis is an immunological disease?

A. Recent data have shifted the weight of the evidence toward an immunological mechanism in polyarteritis nodosa. Laboratory parameters which have been noted include hypergammaglobulinemia, positive rheumatoid factor serology, hypocomplementemia in at least certain patients, and the association of hepatitis-B antigen and necrotizing angiitis. Clinically, the favorable response to corticosteroids and immunosuppressive drugs suggests an immunological basis. The fact that methamphetamine abuse may lead to polyarteritis-like lesions implies a hypersensitivity model for the development of this disease.

REF: Alarcon Segovia, D. "The Necrotizing Vasculitides," in Med Clin North Am, 61:2, 241-260, 1977.

117. Q. What is the evidence that suggests the pathogenetic importance of hypertension in the etiology and development of polyarteritis?

A. Hypertension was once considered as being perhaps the single most important factor in the pathogenesis of polyarteritis. Although it is still considered of prime importance in certain instances, the role of immunologic factors has become increasingly relevant. The lines of evidence suggesting hypertension to be pathogenetically important are the development of polyarteritis-like lesions in the pulmonary vasculature in patients with pulmonary hypertension, and the polyarteritis-like lesions in the mesenteric vasculature in patients who are operated on for coarctation of the aorta.

REF: Alarcon Segovia, D. "The necrotizing vasculitides." in Med Clin North Am, 61:2, 241-260, 1977.

118. Q. Describe the classical pattern of Wegener's granulomatosis.

A. This disorder presents generally with necrotizing granulomatous involvement of the upper and lower respiratory tract. Necrotizing vasculitis is invariably present, and focal glomerulonephritis may frequently be seen. Central nervous system disease may develop as well as sinusitis and polysystemic disease.

REF: Alarcon Segovia, D. "The necrotizing vasculitides," in Med Clin North Am, 61:2, 241-260, 1977.

119. Q. Discuss the concept of limited forms of Wegener's granulomatosis.

A. Wegener's granulomatosis may present as pulmonary involvement, occasionally in an asymptomatic form with the diagnosis being established by biopsy following a routine chest radiograph. Renal disease and multisystemic features are generally absent. However, the course may be variable and subsequent dissemination of the disease may occur. Similarly, the response to treatment may also be somewhat variable, although as a general rule the limited form of the disease is milder and more responsive to treatment than is the disseminated form. Involvement of the eye has been described as another variant of limited Wegener's granulomatosis.

REF: Coutu, R. E. , Klein, M. , Lessell, S. , et. al. "Limited form of Wegener's granulomatosis." JAMA 233:8, 868-871, 1975.

Israel, H. L. and Patchefsky, A. S. "Wegener's granulomatosis of lung: Diagnosis and treatment." Ann Intern Med 74, 881-891, 1971.

120. Q. What are the "variants" of Wegener's granulomatosis that are currently recognized?

A. In addition to the limited forms of Wegener's granulomatosis usually involving the lung, there are two other serious disorders which are felt to belong to the spectrum of Wegener's. These include lethal midline granuloma and pseudotumor of the orbit.

REF: Alacron Segovia, D. "The necrotizing vasculitides," in Med Clin North Am, 61:2, 241-260, 1977.

121. Q. Discuss the treatment of Wegener's granulomatosis.

A. Although corticosteroid drugs have been extensively used in the treatment of this disorder, it appears from some long-term following data that perhaps cyclophosphamide may be the drug of choice in this disease, either given alone or in combination with corticosteroid drugs. Other immunosuppressive medication has also been given with encouraging results such as methotrexate as well as azathioprine. However, cyclophosphamide has achieved perhaps the largest following.

REF: Reza, M. J. , Dornfeld, L. , Goldberg, L. S. , et. al. Wegener's granulomatosis." Arth Rheum 18:5, 501-506, 1975.

122. Q. Comment on the long-term prognosis with cyclophosphamide in the treatment of Wegener's granulomatosis.

A. The disease remains potentially fatal and no certain improvement can be expected in all cases. However, in a study of ten patients with Wegener's granulomatosis treated with cyclophosphamide and followed for periods up to 7 years, it was noted that six patients have remained in complete remission for a mean duration of 38 months. The long-term effectiveness of cyclophosphamide in this disease appears promising and in some cases long range remissions may occur.

REF: Reza, M.J., Dornfeld, L., Goldberg, L.S., et. al. "Wegener's granulomatosis." Arth Rheum 18:5, 501-506, 1975.

123. Q. What are the pathological criteria enabling a histological diagnosis of Wegener's granulomatosis?

A. Necrotizing granulomatous lesions of the upper and lower respiratory tract or of the sinuses associated with generalized necrotizing angiitis constitute the tissue diagnosis of Wegener's granulomatosis. In addition, renal involvement with a necrotizing focal glomerulonephritis may be seen in disseminated cases.

REF: Boyle, J.A. and Buchanan, W.W. "Clinical Rheumatology." Blackwell Scientific Publications, Oxford and Edinburgh, 1971, p. 532.

124. Q. What is generally the cause of death in patients with Wegener's granulomatosis?

A. In general when patients die from this disorder, they succumb to pulmonary insufficiency, which may be aggravated by concomitant bronchopneumonia, and renal failure. Central nervous system disease may also occur and lead to a fatal outcome, but this occurs somewhat less frequently.

REF: Boyle, J.A. and Buchanan, W.W. "Clinical Rheumatology." Blackwell Scientific Publications, Oxford and Edinburgh, 1971, p. 533.

125. Q. What would be your treatment for a patient with relatively good renal function who is acutely ill and perhaps dying with extensive pulmonary hemorrhaging from Goodpasture's syndrome?

A. This area remains controversial and without sufficiently reliable clinical data to form definitive conclusions.

In general, two choices appear relatively feasible. The first is the intravenous administration of massive doses of corticosteroid drugs, while the second is bilateral nephrectomy with renal transplantation of a compatible donor kidney. Both procedures have been reported as being successful in inducing the cessation of pulmonary hemorrhage.

REF: Torrente, A., Popovitzer, M.M., Guggenheim, S.J., and Schrier, R.W. "Serious pulmonary hemorrhage, glomerulonephritis, and massive steroid therapy." Ann Intern Med 83, 218-219, 1975.

Nowakowski, A., Grove, R.B., King, L.H., JR., et.al. "Goodpasture's syndrome: recovery from severe pulmonary hemorrhage after bilateral nephrectomy." Ann Intern Med 75, 243-250, 1971.

126. Q. Although the etiology of Goodpasture's syndrome is of course not known, discuss the current concepts of pathogenesis.

A. In several instances, the exposure to hydrocarbon fumes has been held to be an important issue. In one study, five out of six patients who developed Goodpasture's syndrome had a history of heavy hydrocarbon exposure. Similarly, genetic factors are deemed to be of significance, perhaps in combination with an environmental factor. Viral and bacterial factors have also been considered, and Goodpasture's original case reported in 1919 followed an influenza infection.

REF: D'Apice, A.J.F., Kincaid Smith, P., Becker, G.J., et.al. "Goodpasture's syndrome in identical twins." Ann Intern Med 88:1, 61-62, 1978.

Beirne, G.J. "Goodpasture's syndrome and exposure to solvents." JAMA 222, 1555, 1972.

127. Q. Discuss the spectrum of disorders in the Wegener's granulomatosis group including lymphomatoid granulomatosis and lethal midline granuloma.

A. Wegener's granulomatosis is defined by the presence of a necrotizing angiitis and granulomatous inflammation involving the lungs, upper airways, and the kidneys. It is responsive to cytotoxic agents and perhaps to corticosteroid medication. Both generalized and limited forms may occur, the latter restricted to either the lung or the upper airway region.

Although lethal midline granuloma may be considered an independent disorder, many authorities believe it to be a variant of Wegener's granulomatosis. Lymphomatoid granulomatosis, on the other hand, is characterized by atypical necrotic lymphoreticular infiltrates with not infrequent cutaneous and neurologic involvement. Responsiveness to treatment is poor and the outcome is generally fatal. Another recently described category within this spectrum is that of benign lymphocytic angiitis and granulomatosis. This condition is regularly responsive to chlorambucil and is typified by nodular lesions composed of mature lymphocytes and plasma cells.

REF: Israel, H. L., Patchefsky, A. S., and Saldana, M. J. "Wegener's granulomatosis, lymphomatoid granulomatosis, and benign lymphocytic angiitis and granulomatosis of lung." Ann Intern Med 87, 691-699, 1977.

128. Q. Discuss the current concepts of treatment in Goodpasture's syndrome.

A. This syndrome of hemorrhagic pulmonary disease and glomerulonephritis remains a frequently fatal disorder. Various forms of treatment have been advocated, none with consistently favorable results. Nephrectomy has been advised for pulmonary hemorrhaging, as well as immunosuppressive medication such as nitrogen mustard, azathioprine, and corticosteroid medication. Anticoagulant medication has been a subject of controversy, but may decrease intravascular fibrin formation in the glomerulus.

REF: Whitworth, J. A., Lawrence, J. R., Meadows, R. "Goodpasture's syndrome: a review of nine cases and an evaluation of therapy." Aust NZ J Med 4, 167-177, 1974.

129. Q. Mixed cryoglobulinemia may be found in which types of disorders?

A. An idiopathic variety of mixed cryoglobulinemia may be seen. However, in addition, various other disorders may give rise to cryoglobulins of the IgM and IgG type. These include various infections, connective tissue disorders such as systemic lupus erythematosus, lymphoproliferative disorders, and inflammatory liver disease.

REF: Levo, Y., Gorevic, P. D., Kassab, H. J., et. al. "Liver involvement in the syndrome of mixed cryoglobulinemia." Ann Intern Med 87, 287-292, 1977.

130. Q. Describe the typical clinical features of essential mixed cryoglobulinemia.

A. The clinical triad of purpura, arthralgias, and weakness has traditionally described this syndrome. Systemic vasculitis occurs almost invariably involving the kidneys with an immune complex glomerulonephritis which may be a cause of death. Hepatosplenomegaly and liver dysfunction may be seen. The latter may be related in part to Hepatitis-B virus exposure in up to two thirds of patients.

REF: Levo, Y. , Gorevic, P.D. , Kassab, H.J. , et.al. "Liver involvement in the syndrome of mixed cryoglobulinemia." Ann Intern Med 87, 287-292, 1977.

131. Q.   Describe the myopathy that may be seen in the course of Sjogren's syndrome.

A.   Muscular pain, weakness, and atrophy may be seen in Sjogren's syndrome.   Elevation of the muscle enzymes in serum as well as electromyographic changes similar to those seen in polymyositis may be present.   The histopathological pattern seen on muscle biopsy features degenerative changes in muscle fibers as well as interstitial inflammatory cells.   Perhaps of specific diagnostic importance is the presence quite frequently of what are said to be characteristic microcystic changes in the muscle fibers.

REF: Denko, C. W. and Old, J. W. "Myopathy in the sicca syndrome (Sjogren's syndrome)." <u>Am J Clin Path</u> 51:5, 631-637, 1969.

132. Q.   What is the relationship of beta2 microglobulin concentrations in serum and salivary secretions to Sjogren's syndrome?

A.   Serum concentrations of this protein are elevated in patients with Sjogren's syndrome.   This is especially true of patients with the complications of renal disease or malignant lymphoma.   Salivary concentrations of beta$_2$ microglobulin are elevated in proportion to the degree of lymphocytic infiltration and thus may provide a useful non-invasive technique for the quantification of this type of auto-immune inflammation.

REF: Michalski, J. P. , Daniels, T. E. , Talal, N, and Grey, H. M. "Beta2 microglobulin and lymphocytic infiltration in Sjogren's syndrome." <u>N Engl J Med</u> 293:24, 1228-1231, 1975.

133. Q.   Describe the diagnostic features of Sjogren's syndrome.

A.   Sjogren's syndrome is defined by a triad of keratoconjunctivitis sicca, xerostomia, and a connective tissue disorder such as rheumatoid arthritis which is present in perhaps 50% of patients.   The diagnosis is made whenever

any two of these three major features occur. In addition to
rheumatoid arthritis, other types of connective tissue disorders have been described in association with Sjogren's
syndrome. These include systemic lupus erythematosus,
polyarteritis, dermatomyositis, and scleroderma.

REF: Cummings, N.A., Shall, G.L., Asofsky, R.,
Anderson, L.G., and Talal, N. "Sjogren's syndrome -
Newer aspects of research, diagnosis, and therapy." Ann
Intern Med 75:937-950, 1971.

134. Q. Describe the association of Sjogren's syndrome
with pseudolymphoma.

A. The term "pseudolymphoma" refers to lesions
that resemble tumor-like proliferations of lymphoid cells
which do not meet the conventional histological criteria for
malignancy. In general, patients present with striking lymphadenopathy, hepatosplenomegaly, pulmonary infiltrates,
progressive pulmonary insufficiency, deteriorating renal
disease, and elevations of serum macroglobulin concentrations.

REF: Cummings, N.A., Shall, G.L., Asofsky, R., Anderson, L.G., and Talal, N. "Sjogren's syndrome - Newer
aspects of research, diagnosis, and therapy." Ann Intern
Med 75:937-950, 1971.

135. Q. What are the most commonly found malignancies
with Sjogren's syndrome?

A. Patients with Sjogren's syndrome, with or without
the "pseudolymphomatous" complication, may develop frank-
ly malignant lesions. The most common of these are retic-
ulum cell sarcoma, various poorly differentiated lymphomas,
and Waldenstrom's macroglobulinemia.

REF: Cummings, N.A., Shall, G.L., Asofsky, R., Anderson, L.G., and Talal, N. "Sjogren's syndrome - Newer
aspects of research, diagnosis, and therapy." Ann Intern
Med 75:937-950, 1971.

136. Q. Describe the association of Sjogren's syndrome with the HLA system and comment on its significance.

A. Sjogren's syndrome has been associated with HLA-B8 in 50% of patients as compared to a control of 21%. However, there was no correlation between the presence of the HLA-B8 antigen and various functional and clinical parmeters such as salivary flow rates, keratoconjunctivitis sicca, and so forth. It has been suggested that the HLA-B8 antigen is linked to an immune-response gene such that patients with this antigen are more susceptible to the development of immunological phenomena, which are then modified by various environmental or infectious influences.

REF: Fye, K.H., Terasaki, P.I., Moutsopoulos, H., et.al. "Association of Sjogren's syndrome with HLA-B8." Arth Rheum 19.5, 883-886, 1976.

137. Q. Aside from the various connective tissue disorders, what additional diseases are associated with Sjogren's syndrome?

A. Chronic active hepatitis, Hashimoto's thyroiditis, pernicious anemia, interstitial nephritis, renal tubular acidosis, and nephrogenic diabetes insipidus have all been associated with Sjogren's syndrome.

REF: Cipoletti, J.F., Buckingham, R.B., Barnes, E.L., et.al. "Sjogren's syndrome in progressive systemic sclerosis." Ann Intern Med 87, 535-541, 1977.

138. Q. Discuss the neurological manifestations of sarcoidosis.

A. In general, the estimated frequency of neurological sarcoidosis is 5%. Although neurological involvement may be the presenting symptom, widespread evidence of sarcoidosis is often present. Central nervous system involvement occurs in the early stages, while peripheral nerve and muscle involvement is a relatively late finding. Infiltration of the basal structures by a granulomatous meningitis is the most common pathogenesis of symptoms.

REF: Delaney, P. "Neurologic manifestations in sarcoidosis." Ann Intern Med 87:336-345, 1977.

139. Q. What is the prognosis and effect of treatment in neurological sarcoidosis?

A. Corticosteroid medication is the generally accepted treatment. The results are, however, very unpredictable. Transient and chronic courses may occur. Peripheral and muscular involvement appears to respond better to treatment than does central nervous system disease.

REF: Delaney, P. " Neurologic manifestations in sarcoidosis." Ann Intern Med 87:336-345, 1977.

140. Q. Describe the characteristics of T and B lymphocytes in active and inactive sarcoidosis.

A. In patients with active disease, the total number of lymphocytes is reduced as is the number of T lymphocytes. Phytohemagglutinin response was also noted to be depressed. However, patients in remission from their disease showed no differences either in total lymphocyte count, number of T lymphocytes, or phytohemagglutinin responsiveness.

REF: Daniele, R. P. , Rowlands, D. T. , Jr. "Lymphocyte subpopulations in sarcoidosis: Correlation with disease activity and duration." Ann Intern Med 85:953-600, 1976.

141. Q. Discuss the present concepts of leukocyte dysfunction in sarcoidosis.

A. In a study of 20 patients with sarcoidosis, 19 patients tested demonstrated a defect of leukocyte function.
In general this appeared to be due to a chemotactic factor
inactivator in the serum of patients with sarcoidosis. It
has been speculated that perhaps this type of leukocyte defect may in part be responsible for the demonstrable high
frequency of chronic infectious problems in these patients
which include serious fungal, nocardial, myocobacterial,
and viral disorders.

REF: Maderazo, E.G., Ward, P.A., Woronick, C.L.,
et. al. "Leukocyte dysfunction in sarcoidosis." Ann Intern
Med 84, 414-419, 1976.

142. Q. In what other nonrheumatic disorders has chemotactic factor inactivator been found in high levels?

A. The data suggest that cirrhosis and Hodgkin's disease are associated with unusually high levels of chemotactic
factor inactivator. These levels are higher than those seen
in sarcoidosis, and may account for the increased rate of
infectious complications seen in these diseases.

REF: Maderazo, E.G., Ward, P.A., and Woronick, C.L.,
et. al. "Leukocyte dysfunction in sarcoidosis." Ann Intern
Med 84, 414-419, 1976.

143. Q. Discuss the type and frequency of pleural involvement in sarcoidosis.

A. Although pulmonary involvement is a well recognized complication of sarcoidosis, pleural involvement with
or without effusions is distinctly a rare event. Nonetheless,
there have been well documented reports of pleural involvement with noncaseating granulomata with or without effusion. The diagnosis must be based on histological demonstration of the granulomatous lesions characteristic of
sarcoidosis. Appropriate exclusions of such potential problems as chronic granulomatous infections, tuberculosis, and
so forth, are of course essential to the diagnosis.

REF: Beekman, J. F., Zimmet, S. M., Chun, B. K., and Miranda, A. A. "Spectrum of pleural involvement in sarcoidosis." Arch Intern Med 136, 323-330, 1976.

144. Q. Discuss the types of renal involvement that may be seen in sarcoidosis.

A. Renal involvement is relatively rare in sarcoidosis. However, it does occur and may take the form of one of three presentations. Interstitial nephritis may be seen with granulomata of the renal parenchyma. With increased sensitivity to vitamin D, disorders of calcium homeostasis may be seen and may result in renal disease. Finally, isolated renal disease due to granulomatous involvement may be seen as an isolated event, without significant peripheral sarcoidosis.

REF: King, B. P., Esparza, A. R., Kahn, S. I. and Garella, S. "Sarcoid granulomatous nephritis occurring as isolated renal failure." Arch Intern Med 136, 241-245, 1976.

145. Q. A relatively recent addition to the diagnostic procedures available in sarcoidosis has been the technique of transbroncial lung biopsy. Discuss the merits and relative risks of this procedure in sarcoidosis.

A. The chief problem with transbronchial lung biopsy is the threat of hemorrhage, and careful hematologic screening, including prothrombin time and bleeding time should be obtained prior to the procedure. However, the general risk of morbidity is quite acceptable, and the avoidance of general anesthesia a definite benefit. The diagnostic yield is on the order of 63% which is equivalent to that obtained by liver biopsy. Hence, the procedure appears to be a useful one in certain cases where more direct confirmation of the diagnosis is lacking.

REF: Koontz, C. H., Joyner, L. R., Nelson, R. A., "Trans bronchial lung biopsy via the fiberoptic bronchoscope in sarcoidosis." Ann Intern Med 85, 64-66, 1976.

146. Q. What is the status of the Kveim test in the diagnosis of sarcoidosis?

A. The Kveim test depends on purity of the antigen and this is not always easily assured. Additionally, some question has been raised about the specificity of the Kveim test. In the latter stages of disease, its reliability has been questioned. Therefore, the disease is often confirmed by techniques other than the Kveim test which is not readily available to most physicians. Tissue diagnosis remains the most reliable means of a specific diagnosis.

REF: Koerner, S. K., Sakowitz, A. J., Appelman, R. I., et. al. "Transbronchial lung biopsy for the diagnosis of sarcoidosis." New Engl J Med 293:6, 268-270, 1975.

147. Q. Discuss the clinical features of sarcoidosis that would allow a physician to make the diagnosis on a clinical basis pending biopsy or tissue confirmation.

A. Sarcoidosis has been defined clinically as a chronic granulomatous disorder of uncertain etiology involving the peripheral and mediastinal lymph nodes, liver, spleen, lungs, eyes, parotid glands, and the bones and joints. Skin tests, including the tuberculin test, are frequently nonreactive. The laboratory findings suggestive of the disorder include hypercalciuria and hypergammaglobulinemia.

REF: Scully, R. E., Galdabini, J. J., and McNeely, B. U. "Case records of the Massachusetts General Hospital." New Engl J Med 293:22, 1138-1145, 1975.

148. Q. The histological parameters defining sarcoidosis are the presence of granulomatous lesions with epithelioid cells, giant cells, and lacking significant necrosis. Discuss the differential diagnosis of such lesions and the important exclusions to the histological verification of this disease.

A. Various fungal disorders and tuberculosis must be carefully excluded before a tissue diagnosis of sarcoidosis is made. Therefore, acid fast and fungal stains are important as well as cultures for these organisms. Beryllium and local sarcoid tissue reactions must also be excluded. Therefore, when noncaseating granulomata are seen in lymph nodes, spleen, liver, or in the pulmonary tissues, and careful exclusion of chronic fungal disorders and tuberculosis is accomplished, then a tissue diagnosis of sarcoidosis may be rendered.

REF: Scully, R.E., Galdabini, J.J., and McNeely, B.U. "Case records of the Massachusetts General Hospital." New Engl J Med 293:22, 1138-1145, 1975.

149. Q. Discuss the types of cardiac involvement seen in sarcoidosis.

A. Pericardial involvement has been noted. The root of the aorta may be affected, and papillary muscle disease may lead to mitral regurgitation. Ventricular septal disease may lead to conduction abnormalities. Granulomatous lesions and fibrosis of the myocardium may lead to a cardiomyopathy and to cor pulmonale.

REF: Scully, R.E., Galdabini, J.J., and McNeely, B.U. "Case records of the Massachusetts General Hospital." New Engl J Med 293:22, 1138-1145, 1975.

150. Q. When a physician is faced with pulmonary sarcoidosis, what are the current concepts of treatment with corticosteroid medication?

A. No convincing clinical data have yet emerged to build a case for corticosteroid medication in the treatment of pulmonary sarcoidosis. The fact that many clinicians utilize steroid drugs depends on anecdotal evidence that these medications offer significant benefit. Whether they prevent pulmonary fibrosis, pulmonary hypertension, and the development of progressive pulmonary disease is an undecided issue. However, it is generally accepted that treatment with systemic corticosteroid drugs is indicated in any patient with confirmed pulmonary sarcoidosis with significant dyspnea.

REF: Sarcoidosis, Medical staff conference, University of California, San Francisco, West J Med 126, 288-296, 1977.

151. Q. Describe the typical erosions seen radiographically in the hands in sarcoidosis.

A. Occasionally sarcoidosis may cause diagnostic
confusion between gout and rheumatoid arthritis. All three
disorders may produce erosive lesions in the hands. However, the typical erosion of sarcoidosis may be distinguish-
ed by several characteristic features. In general, the erosions of sarcoidosis tend to affect the distal phalanx and
appear centrally just beneath the subarticular bone.

REF: Boyle, J.A. and Buchanan, W.W., "Clinical Rheumatology." Blackwell Scientific Publications, Oxford and
Edinburgh, 1971, p. 237.

VIII.   POLYMYALGIA RHEUMATICA AND GIANT CELL ARTERITIS

152.   Q.   What are the most important diagnostic features of polymyalgia rheumatica?

A.   Polymyalgia rheumatica may be defined by the presence of persistent proximal muscular pain and stiffness, in a patient of 55 years or more, with a sedimentation rate in excess of 50 mm/hr.   In general, treatment with relatively low doses of corticosteroid medication results in a prompt improvement in symptoms.

REF: Fauchald, P., Rygvold, O., Oystese, B. "Temporal arteritis and polymyalgia rheumatica.   Clinical and biopsy findings." Ann Intern Med 77:845-852, 1972.

153.   Q.   What are the systemic complications that may be seen in the polymyalgia rheumatica - giant cell arteritis syndrome?

A.   Systemic involvement may include fatigue, weight loss, fever, headache, anemia, arthralgias with occasionally articular swelling, visual impairment including blindness, vasculitis not only of the temporal arteries, but also of the vertebral, subclavian, carotid, axillary, brachial, iliac, femoral, popliteal, coronary, and mesenteric arteries, as well as liver involvement and central nervous system disease.

REF: Healey, L.A., Parker, F., Wilske, K.R. "Polymyalgia rheumatica and giant cell arteritis." Arth Rheum 12: 138-141, 1971.

154.   Q.   Describe the type of liver involvement that has been described in association with polymyalgia rheumatica and giant cell arteritis.

A.   Abnormalities of liver function have been frequently described in patients with the polymyalgia rheumatica - giant cell arteritis syndrome.   These include elevation of the transaminase levels as well as the alkaline phosphatase and increased retention of bromsulphalein.   Liver biopsy material has yielded inconsistent findings. However, several reports have now appeared describing granulomatous hepatic infiltrates in both polymyalgia rheumatica and giant cell arteritis. Treatment with corticosteroid medication resulted in prompt improvement in liver function abnormalities.

REF: Litwack, K. D. , Bohan, A. , and Silverman, L. "Granulomatous liver disease and giant cell arteritis. Case report and literature review." Journal of Rheumat 4:3, 307-312, 1977.

155. Q. What are the clinical features of giant cell granulomatous angiitis of the central nervous system?

     A. Granulomatous arteritis of the central nervous system may occur either as an isolated event or in association with evidence of temporal giant cell arteritis. Mental changes are associated with evidence of paresis, extrapyramidal signs, visual disorders, involvement of the brainstem, and coma.

REF: Jellinger, K. "Giant cell granulomatous angiitis of the central nervous system." J Neruol 215, 175-190, 1977.

156. Q. What are the typical histological changes seen in a biopsy of the temporal artery in a patient with temporal arteritis?

     A. The histological picture of temporal arteritis includes infiltration of the entire wall of the blood vessel with inflammatory cells which typically feature large numbers of giant cells. Other commonly observed features are those of intimal proliferation and thrombosis. Of importance is the fact that these histological abnormalities may occur in a patchy distribution with "skip" areas where entirely normal histology may be contiguous with severely diseased tissue.

REF: Fauchald, P. , Rygvold, O. , Oystese, B. "Temporal arteritis and polymyalgia rheumatica. Clinical and biopsy findings." Ann Intern Med 77:845-852, 1972.

157. Q. Describe the pathogenesis of visual blindness in temporal arteritis.

A. Visual impairment, including complete blindness, has been well described in patients with temporal arteritis. This may occur with or without the syndrome of polymyalgia rheumatica. Arteritis with occlusion of a branch of the central retinal artery may result in blindness. However, more commonly visual impairment is due to ischemic optic neuritis. Once it occurs, blindness is usually irreversible.

REF: Goodman, M. A. , Pearson, C. M. "Polymyalgia rheumatica and associated arteritis: a review." Calif Med 111: 453-460, 1969.

158. Q. Discuss the probability of corticosteroid withdrawal in a patient with polymyalgia rheumatica and comment on abrupt as opposed to gradual steroid withdrawal.

A. Although polymyalgia rheumatica may be a self-limited disease, it can also require long-term corticosteroid administration for periods of five years and longer. In a study of 18 patients, prednisolone withdrawal was attempted by either an abrupt or gradual method. There were no significant differences noted between either method of withdrawal, and cessation of corticosteroid treatment was not possible in these patients.

REF: Esselinckx, W. , Doherty, S. M. , and Dixon, A.ST.J. "Polymyalgia rheumatica. Abrupt and gradual withdrawal of prednisolone treatment, clinical and laboratory observations." Ann Rheum Dis 36:219-224, 1977.

159. Q. What is the usefulness of temporal arteriography in the diagnosis of temporal arteritis?

A. Superficial temporal arteriography provides a very sensitive, although perhaps a somewhat nonspecific, tool to detect abnormalities of the temporal artery. Almost all patients with temporal arteritis have abnormal temporal arteriography. However, arteriosclerotic abnormalities may cause confusion and result in false positive arteriographic findings. The technique is most useful when classical changes are noted on the arteriograph such as diffuse areas of constriction, obstruction, and dilatation.

REF: Horwitz, H.M., Pepe, P.F., Johnsrude, I.S., et. al. "Temporal arteriography and immunofluorescence as diagnostic tools in temporal arteritis." J Rheum 4:1, 76-85, 1977.

IX. THE HLA HISTOCOMPATIBILITY COMPLEX
AND RELATED DISORDERS (ANKYLOSING
SPONDYLITIS AND REITER'S SYNDROME)

160. Q. Describe the genetics of the HLA system in human
beings.

A. There are four loci on the sixth chromosome
named A, B, C, and D. The A and B loci are most commonly tested for and are co-dominant alleles. The C locus appears to be of little importance and has but a few
alleles. The D locus represents the mixed lymphocyte
culture response. Since each individual has two sixth-
chromosomes, four potentially different HLA specificities
can be inherited. An offspring will thus have one sixth-
chromosome or two HLA antigens in common with each
parent.

REF: Kemple, K. and Bluestone, R. "The Histocompatibility Complex and Rheumatic Diseases." <u>Med Clin North
Am</u>, 61:2, 331-345, March 1977.

161. Q. What other loci are associated with the histocompatibility complex?

A. Complement components, properdin factor B,
beta-2 microglobulins, and possibly immune-response
genes.

REF: Kemple, K. and Bluestone, R. "The Histocompatibility Complex and Rheumatic Diseases." <u>Med Clin North
Am</u>, 61:2, 331-345, March 1977.

162. Q. What is meant by "linkage disequilibrium?"

A. Each allele will occur at a frequency that is independent of other associated alleles. To the extent that a
given allele occurs at either a greater or a lesser frequency
than expected from individual frequencies, then that allele
is said to be in "linkage disequilibrium."

REF: Kemple, K. and Bluestone, R. "The Histocompatibility Complex and Rheumatic Diseases." <u>Med Clin North
Am</u>, 61:2, 331-345, March 1977.

163. Q. Which diseases have been associated with an
increased frequency of HLA-B8?

A. Dermatitis herpetiformis (58%), celiac disease
(78%), myasthenia gravis (52%), Graves' Disease (47%),
and chronic active hepatitis (68%).

REF: Kemple, K. and Bluestone, R. "The Histocompatibility Complex and Rheumatic Diseases." Med Clin North
Am, 61:2, 331-345, 1977.

164. Q. What are the relative frequencies of the HLA-B27
antigen in the Caucasian population; in American Blacks, in
ankylosing spondylitis; in Reiter's syndrome; in psoriatic
arthritis with spondylitis; in juvenile chronic polyarthritis
with sacroiliitis; in ulcerative colitis with spondylitis; in
Crohn's disease with spondylitis; and in Yersinia arthritis?

A. In the normal Caucasian population the HLA-B27
antigen is found in 6-8%; it is 4% in American Blacks; in
ankylosing spondylitis 91%; in Reiter's syndrome 79%; in
psoriatic arthritis with spondylitis 50%; in juvenile chronic
polyarthritis with sacroiliitis 84%; in colitic spondylitis 75%;
in Crohn's disease with spondylitis 30%; and in Yersinia
arthritis 90%.

REF: Wright, V., Sturrock, R.D., and Dick, W.C. "Seronegative Spondarthritides." In "Recent Advances in Rheumatology." Edited by W. Watson Buchanan and W. Carson Dick,
Churchill Livingstone, 1976, 193-215.

165. Q. Discuss the postulated mechanisms by which the
HLA-B27 antigen might influence the development of ankylosing spondylitis, Reiter's syndrome, and other
spondyloarthritides.

A. It has been theorized that the HLA-B27 antigen
could serve as a molecular receptor for some infective organism such as a virus, bacteria, or other as yet unknown
agent. Alternatively, there could be common antigenicity
between the HLA-B27 antigen and antigens that are a part of
infecting organisms. If this were the case, then an immune
response directed at the invading organisms would also be

directed against the HLA-B27 antigen present in selected
tissues such as the fibroblasts and mesenchymal components in spinal ligamentous structures, sacroiliac joints,
and peripheral joints. However, perhaps the most attrac-
tive hypothesis at this time is the one that implicates a linkage disequilibrium between the HLA-B27 antigen and an immune-response gene so that certain abnormalities in immunological reactivity occurring as a response to an infective
agent would then give rise to the clinical expression of disease. An animal model for this hypothesis is the lymphocytic choriomeningitis virus which can infect all mice; but
only certain mice with an abnormal immune-response gene
allowing for serologic and lymphocytic hyper-reactivity
subsequently develop clinical disease.

REF: Kemple, K. and Bluestone, R. "The Histocompatibility Complex and Rheumatic Diseases." Med Clin North
Am, 61:2, 331-345, March 1977.

166. Q. Discuss the diagnostic criteria for ankylosing
spondylitis.

A. The definitive diagnosis of ankylosing spondylitis
does not depend on the HLA-B27 antigen, which is usually
positive, but may be negative in up to 10% of patients. Instead, the diagnosis depends on radiographic evidence of
bilateral sacroiliitis with one of the clinical criteria listed
below, or the presence of unilateral sacroiliitis with two of
the clinical criteria. These clinical criteria include:
(a) Limitation of lumbar spine motion in three planes, flexion, extension, lateral flexion. (b) Pain in the lumbar spine
or in the dorsolumbar junction. (c) Limitation of chest expansion to 2.5 cm or less when measured at the level of the
fourth intercostal space.

REF: Bennett, P.H. and Burch, T.A. "New York Sympo-
sium on population studies in rheumatic diseases. New
diagnostic criteria." Bull Rheum Dis, 17:453, 1967.

167. Q. Describe the extra-skeletal manifestations of
ankylosing spondylitis.

A. Anterior uveitis of the nongranulomatous type
may occur in up to 25% of patients, and may antedate the

development of spondylitis. It appears to be more common
in patients with peripheral joint involvement and in HLA-B27
positive individuals. Cardiopulmonary manifestations include heart block, aortic insufficiency, cardiomegaly, pericarditis, and apical pulmonary fibrosis. Amyloidosis may
occur with chronic cases. A rare manifestation is
involvement of the cauda equina.

REF: Engleman, E. G. and Engleman, E. P. "Ankylosing
Spondylitis. Recent Advances in Diagnosis and Treatment."
Med Clin North Am, 61:2, 347-364, March 1977.

168. Q. Compare and contrast the clinical and radiographic
features of ankylosing spondylitis, Reiter's syndrome, psoriatic arthritis, and arthritis with inflammatory bowel
disease.

A. Sacroiliitis occurs early in the course of ankylosing spondylitis, but is seen in only 20% of patients with
these other types of spondyloarthritides. In ankylosing
spondylitis and in colitic arthritis, the sacroiliitis is symmetrical and the syndesmophytes are of the "marginal"
type. In psoriatic arthritis and Reiter's syndrome, sacroiliitis is frequently assymetric and syndesmophytes are of
the non-marginal type. Larger joints are involved with colitic arthritis and ankylosing spondylitis, with a predilection
for the lower extremities in the latter disease. Small and
large joints are involved in both psoriatic arthritis and
Reiter's syndrome, with a predeliction for the upper extremity in the former and the lower extremity in the latter.

REF: McEwen, C., Di Tata, D., Lingg, C., et. al. "Ankylosing spondylitis and spondylitis accompanying ulcerative
colitis, regional enteritis, psoriasis, and Reiter's disease."
Arthritis Rheum, 14:391, 1971.

169. Q. What genetic counseling would you give a patient
known to be positive for the HLA-B27 antigen?

A. It is estimated that approximately 20% of HLA-B27
positive individuals either have or will develop one of the
spondyloarthritides such as ankylosing spondylitis. In the
first degree relatives, if an individual is B27 positive then

there is a 50% chance that ankylosing spondylitis will develop; while if he is B27 negative, there is a 21% chance of developing the disease. There is little clinical difference between +B27 and -B27 individuals with ankylosing spondylitis, although anterior uveitis appears to be more common in the former than in the latter.

REF: Brewerton, D. A. "HLA-B27 and the inheritance of susceptibility to rheumatic diseases." Arth Rheum, 19:656, 1976.

170. Q. Discuss the previously held opinions as to the prevalence and sex distribution of ankylosing spondylitis and compare these to current concepts that have emerged out of studies with the HLA-B27 antigenic marker.

A. Traditional estimates as to the prevalence of ankylosing spondylitis in the Caucasian population were on the order of 0.1% with a male:female ratio of 10:1. However, in recent studies with "healthy" blood donors, it was found that 20% of B27 positive individuals met the clinical and radiographic criteria for a definitive diagnosis of ankylosing spondylitis. The male:female ratio was equal. Therefore, it would appear that the true estimate as to the prevalence of ankylosing spondylitis is on the order of 1%, or 10-fold greater than had been previously assumed. Furthermore, there are as many women affected as there are men, although it would appear that men tend to express their disease in a more obvious clinical fashion than women.

REF: Calin, A., and Fries, J. F. "The striking prevalence of ankylosing spondylitis in "healthy" B27 positive males and females. A controlled study." New Eng J Med, 293, 835, 1975.

171. Q. In addition to the HLA-B27 antigen which is usually positive in ankylosing spondylitis, what are the other laboratory features that are characteristic of this disorder?

A. Although the acute phase reactants appear to be generally normal, elevation of the sedimentation rate is seen in 80% of cases. Mild anemia of the hypochromic type is seen in 20-30%. Elevation of the protein in cerebrospinal

fluid may occur, as may elevation in the serum creatine
phosphokinase. Reports of the presence of IgG anti-globulins,
elevated C4 levels, and the presence of immune complexes
have appeared recently. However, in general the rheumatoid factor by traditional methods is negative. T and B cell
typing is normal.

REF: Engleman, E. G. and Engleman, E. P. "Ankylosing
spondylitis. Recent Advances in Diagnosis and Treatment."
Med Clin North Am, 61:2, 347-364, March 1977.

172. Q. What are the typical clinical features of ankylosing
spondylitis?

       A. The insidious onset of low back pain and stiffness
in a young man (or woman) between the ages of 15 and 30
years of age is usually associated with morning stiffness
and nocturnal pain. Peripheral joint involvement may occur
and, in 20% of patients, may antedate spinal involvement.
Restriction of motion in the lumbar spine is in all directions, including flexion, extension, and lateral flexion. Sacroiliac joint tenderness is present in early stages, although
as fusion occurs the sacroiliac joints become non-tender.
Chest expansion is generally limited below 2.5 cm at the
nipple line. Shober's test is usually positive, and flattening of the normal lordotic curve at the lumbar region is
characteristic.

REF: Ogryzlo, M. A. and Rosen, P. S. "Ankylosing (Marie-
Strumpell) spondylitis." Postgrad Med 45:182, 1969.

173. Q. What five questions might you wish to ask your
patients about their symptoms so as to sort out which of
them were likely candidates for ankylosing spondylitis with
the highest degree of sensitivity and specificity?

       A. Four of the following five "spondylitic" responses
predicted the diagnosis of ankylosing spondylitis with 95%
sensitivity and 85% specificity. (1) less than 40 years of
age at onset; (2) insidious onset; (3) at least 3 months

duration; (4) morning back stiffness; (5) improvement in symptoms with exercise.

REF: Calin, A., Porta, J., Schurman, D., et. al. "Comparing HLA-B27 and an appropriate history. A new look at an old perspective." Abst. in "HLA and Disease - Predisposition to Disease and Clinical Implications. Paris, France. June 1976, p. 22.

174. Q. Discuss the current concepts of treatment in ankylosing spondylitis.

A. Antiinflammatory drugs are combined with a program of spondylitic exercises designed to strengthen the extensor muscles of the back. Awareness and attention to proper posture, both while awake and during sleep are of considerable importance. Therapy with nonsteroidal antiinflammatory agents such as indomethacin and phenylbutazone has been the mainstay of treatment. These are generally somewhat more effective than salicylates, although the latter may be of value in selected cases. The newer nonsteroidal antiinflammatory agents such as naproxen, ibuprofen, tolmetin, and others appear to be promising. Gold salts and corticosteroids are of no significant benefit. Radiotherapy to the lumbar spine has been abandoned due to the later appearance of malignant disease. However, in selected cases, localized radiation therapy to a limited portion of the lumbar spine may be of value in terminating severe and otherwise uncontrollable pain.

REF: Calabro, J.J. "An appraisal of the medical and surgical management of ankylosing spondylitis." Clin Orthop Rel Res 60:125, 1968.

175. Q. Discuss the concept of enthesopathy as it relates to ankylosing spondylitis.

A. The term "enthesis" refers to the area of attachment of ligaments to bone. In ankylosing spondylitis, it is hypothesized that persistent inflammation in this area eventually leads to the characteristic findings of ligamentous ossification, formation of syndesmophytes, and bony ankylosis of joints.

REF: Ball, J. "Enthesopathy of rheumatoid and ankylosing spondylitis. Ann Rheum Dis, 30:213, 1971.

176. Q. What lymphocyte abnormalities exist in ankylosing spondylitis?

A. The percentage of T lymphocytes appears to be lower in patients with ankylosing spondylitis. This observation is felt to be due to an increase in "null" cells. There is no correlation between HLA-B27 positivity. Although it has been reported that suboptimal doses of PHA failed to adequately stimulate the lymphocytes of ankylosing spondylitic patients, optimal doses of PHA produced expected levels of lymphocyte responsiveness. Such data are interpreted as suggesting a role for delayed hypersensitivity in ankylosing spondylitis.

REF: Fan, P.T., Clements, P.J., Yu, D.T.Y., et.al. Ann Rheum Dis 36, 471-473, 1977.

177. Q. Comment on mortality rates in patients with ankylosing spondylitis.

A. It is important to separate patients with ankylosing spondylitis who have not been treated with radiation therapy from those who have, because in the latter group there appears to be an increased frequency of various cancers. Nonetheless, even in those patients who have never received radiation therapy, ankylosing spondylitis is associated with increased mortality rates primarily relating to ulcerative colitis, nephritis, tuberculosis, respiratory disorders, cerebrovascular disease, and circulatory diseases.

REF: Radford, E.P., Doll, R., and Smith, P.G. "Mortality among patients with ankylosing spondylitis not given x-ray therapy." New Engl J Med 297:11, 572-576, 1977.

178. Q. What evidence is there to suggest a humoral abnormality in ankylosing spondylitis?

A. It is widely accepted that rheumatoid factors and other serologies are negative in ankylosing spondylitis. However, some evidence of increased levels of immunoglobulins and decreased complement has been reported. Additionally, in a study of 125 patients with ankylosing spondylitis, the majority (60%) demonstrated homogeneous staining antinuclear antibody titers of restricted specificity. These antibodies reacted with leukocytes, occasionally with lymphocytes, but not with nuclear material from other human and nonhuman substrates.

REF: Vasey, F.B. and Kinsella, T.D. "Increased frequency of leukocyte reactive antinuclear antibody in patients with ankylosing spondylitis." J Rheum 4:2, 158-164, 1977.

179. Q. Comment on the relative role of genetic and environmental factors in the pathogenesis of ankylosing spondylitis.

A. With the association of the HLA-B27 antigen with ankylosing spondylitis together with the familial aggregation demonstrated in this disorder, there is little question about the importance of genetic factors in ankylosing spondylitis. However, studies with monozygotic twins have demonstrated disordance for ankylosing spondylitis, suggesting that environmental factors appear to be necessary for the development and ultimate expression of the disease.

REF: Eastmond, C.J. and Woodrow, J.C. "Discordance for ankylosing spondylitis in monozygotic twins." Ann Rheum Dis 36, 360-364, 1977.

180. Q. Discuss the most common causes of a painful heel.

A. Achilles tendinitis and plantar fascitis are the most common causes of a severely painful heel, and they occur principally in Reiter's syndrome and ankylosing spondylitis. As might be expected, men are affected more frequently than women. On the other hand, sub-Achilles bursitis affected women more frequently than men, occurred mostly in rheumatoid arthritis, and rarely resulted in severe talalgia. Calcaneal spurs occurring with degenerative osteoarthritis, rarely produced clinical symptoms.

REF: Gerster, J. C. , Vischer, T. L. , Bennani, A. , and Fallet, G. H. "The painful heel." Ann Rheum Dis 36, 343-348, 1977.

181. Q. What is the relationship between Yersinia arthritis and HLA-B27?

    A. Both HLA-B27 positive and negative individuals develop arthritis following infection with Yersinia. However, in the HLA-B27 positive group, the arthritis tends to be of greater severity, systemic complications such as iritis, conjunctivitis, carditis, and urologic symptoms occur more frequently, and evolution into the complete triad of Reiter's syndrome may be seen. In the HLA-B27 negative group, erythema nodosum is more commonly seen, and the arthritis is of a milder form without systemic complications or progression to Reiter's syndrome.

REF: Laitinen, O. , Leirisalo, M. , and Skylv, G. "Relation between HLA-B27 and clinical features in patients with Yersinia arthritis." Arth Rheum 20:5, 1121-1124, 1977.

182. Q. What is the role of the HLA-B27 antigen in rheumatoid factor negative polyarthritis?

    A. The HLA-B27 antigen is clearly of considerable usefulness in the diagnosis of ankylosing spondylitis and Reiter's syndrome. However, in one large study which attempted to evaluate the role of this antigen in rheumatoid factor negative polyarthritis, it was found that the B27 test was not more helpful than clinical diagnosis. Patients with classical spondyloarthritic syndromes could be separated and appropriately diagnosed by the use of clinical criteria, and the application of the HLA-B27 tissue typing did not improve this process nor did it uncover a subpopulation of patients within the seronegative rheumatoid arthritis group.

REF: Esdaile, J. M. , Dwosh, I. L. , Urowitz, M. B. , et. al. Ann Intern Med 86, 699-702, 1977.

183. Q. What is the association between the arthropathy which follows rubella vaccination and the HLA-B27 antigen?

A. Following both natural rubella infection and immunization with rubella vaccine, there may occur a transient syndrome of polyarthralgias. Although chronic arthritis has not been noted with rubella, vaccination in children may on occasion produce a chronic or recurrent polyarthritis lasting months to even years. Tissue typing techniques have failed to uncover an association between a particular antigen such as B27 and a susceptibility to the development of this type of arthritis.

REF: Griffiths, M.M., Spruance, S.L., Ogra, P.L., et.al. "HLA and recurrent episodic arthropathy associated with rubella vaccination." Arth Rheum 20:6, 1192-1197, 1977.

184. Q. Discuss nongranulomatous anterior uveitis as a marker for ankylosing spondylitis.

A. Patients with ankylosing spondylitis are characterized by a positive HLA-B27 tissue typing, although this is not a prerequisite, and B27 negative patients with ankylosing spondylitis have been well described. Nongranulomatous anterior uveitis has also been associated with the B27 antigen, and clearly ankylosing spondylitis and anterior uveitis may occur together. In a scintigraphic study of the sacroiliac joints in acute anterior uveitis, it was noted that anterior uveitis may serve as a clinical marker of a spondylitic diathesis even when clinical, radiographic, and laboratory parameters, including the HLA-B27 antigen, are all negative.

REF: Russell, A.S., Lentle, B.C., Percy, J.S., and Jackson, F.I. "Scintigraphy of sacroiliac joints in acute anterior uveitis." Ann Intern Med 85, 606-608, 1976.

185. Q. List the disorders associated with HLA-B27 antigen.

A. Ankylosing spondylitis and Reiter's syndrome are most closely linked with the B27 antigen. However, in addition, other disorders which are associated with this antigen include acute anterior uveitis, a subpopulation of juvenile rheumatoid arthritis, psoriatic spondylitis and sacroiliitis, colitic spondylitis and sacroiliitis, and Yersinia arthritis.

REF: Ritzmann, S. E. "HLA patterns and disease associations." JAMA 236:20, 2305-2309, 1976.

186. Q. Is there any evidence that suggests a relationship between the HLA system and systemic lupus erythematosus?

A. The data are not entirely clear on this issue, although there is some suspicion that HLA-B8 and HLA-Bw15 may be associated in a statistically significant fashion with systemic lupus erythematosus.

REF: Ritzmann, S. E. "HLA patterns and disease associations." JAMA 236:20, 2305-2309, 1976.

187. Q. Has Behcet's syndrome been linked to the HLA system?

A. Behcet's syndrome may cause sacroiliitis and has been linked statistically to the HLA-B5 antigen. The data, however, are preliminary in this regard.

REF: Ritzmann, S. E. "HLA patterns and disease associations." JAMA 236:20, 2305-2309, 1976.

188. Q. Describe the clinical and radiographic features of ankylosing hyperostosis (Forestier's disease) of the spine and its association with the HLA-B27 antigen.

A. Forestier's disease of the spine is characterized by proliferative and exuberant new bone formation which assumes a "flowing" pattern on radiographs. The site of ossification is generally along the anterolateral aspect of the vertebrae particularly in the thoracic spine. Large osteophytic formations may be seen in the cervical and lumbar vertebrae at the junctions of the vertebral body and intervertebral disc. New bone growth may also be seen at sites of ligamentous attachment in the pelvic bones, calcaneus, tarsal bones, patella, and so forth. The association with the HLA-B27 antigen is on the order of 34%.

REF: Resnick, D., Linovitz, R. J., and Feingold, M. L. "Postoperative heterotopic ossification in patients with ankylosing hyperostosis of the spine (Forestier's disease)." J Rheum 3:3, 313-320, 1976.

189. Q. Compare ankylosing hyperostosis and ankylosing spondylitis and comment on the proposed role of the HLA-B27 antigen in ossification.

A. Both disorders have increased association with the HLA-B27 antigen. Syndesmophyte formation resulting from ossification of the annulus fibrosis characterizes ankylosing spondylitis, whereas in ankylosing hyperostosis there is more exuberant ossification in a regional fashion. Periosteal proliferation and "whiskering" are common to both disorders and at similar ligamentous sites. Thus in both diseases, there appears to be a basic ossification diathesis, which may be an expression of the presence of the B27 antigen.

REF: Resnick, D., Linovitz, R. J., and Feingold, M. L. "Postoperative heterotopic ossification in patients with ankylosing hyperostosis of the spine (Forestier's disease)." J Rheum 3:3, 313-320, 1976.

190. Q. Discuss an orthopedic surgeon's concerns regarding total hip replacement in ankylosing spondylitis and in ankylosing hyperostosis.

A. In both of these disorders, there appears to be a definite tendency for increased ossification. In total hip replacement, this may become a serious postoperative problem with "re-ankylosis" of the hip limiting postoperative mobility.

REF: Resnick, D., Linovitz, R. J., and Feingold, M. L. "Postoperative heterotopic ossification in patients with ankylosing hyperostosis of the spine (Forestier's disease)." J Rheum 3:3, 313-320, 1976.

191. Q. Describe the various patterns of psoriatic arthritis and comment as to their relative frequencies.

A. A "rheumatoid-like" pattern may be seen in approximately 78% of patients. Distal interphalangeal joint arthritis in general represents somewhat more than 16%, while deforming arthritis occurs in approximately 5% of patients. Skin lesions precede the development of arthritis in the vast majority of patients, although in perhaps 16% the arthritis occurs first. Synchronous onset of joint and skin disease is distinctly uncommon.

REF: Roberts, M. E. T., Wright, V. , Hill, A. G. S. , and Mehra, A. C. "Psoriatic arthritis." Ann Rheum Dis 35, 206-212, 1976.

192. Q. What is the current status of methotrexate in psoriatic arthritis?

A. The clinical effectiveness of methotrexate in psoriatic arthritis both for the skin disease as well as for the arthritic disorder has been well established. However, a small but significant risk of hepatotoxicity has emerged from clinical trials. Hepatotoxicity appears to be greatest when methotrexate is given on a daily basis as opposed to weekly. The intravenous route appears to decrease the risk of hepatotoxicity as opposed to the oral route. Approximately 3% of patients given methotrexate appear to develop evidence of cirrhosis or fibrosis, although it is not yet clear as to the importance of other factors independent of the methotrexate itself. Unfortunately, the development of cirrhosis or hepatic fibrosis may occur without betraying its presence by conventional liver function testing. Liver biopsy, advocated by some, remains controversial as a routine measure.

REF: Weinstein, G. D. "Methotrexate." Ann Intern Med 86, 199-204, 1977.

193. Q. Describe the typical findings of methotrexate-induced pneumonitis.

A. This is generally considered to be a hypersensitivity pneumonitis. It is relatively uncommon. Severe pulmonary involvement may occur with chest radiographs revealing diffuse and extensive involvement. Auscultatory findings may be unimpressive. Eosinophilia is usually present. A response to corticosteroid medication and of course withdrawal of the methotrexate results in prompt improvement.

REF: Weinstein, G. D. "Methotrexate." Ann Intern Med 86, 199-204, 1977.

194. Q. Discuss the etiological factors felt to be of importance in the pathogenesis of nongonococcal urethritis.

A. In a study of both asymptomatic as well as symptomatic individuals, Chlamydia trachomatis was isolated from the urethral cultures of 42% of men with nonspecific, nongonococcal urethritis. Other authors have reported as significant cytomegalovirus, T mycoplasma, Herspesvirus hominis, Trichomonas vaginalis, and other bacteria.

REF: Holmes, K. K., Handsfield, H. H., Wang, S. P., et. al. "Etiology of nongonococcal urethritis." New Engl J Med 292:23, 1199-1204, 1975.

195. Q. Although Reiter's syndrome is generally a disease of favorable prognosis, in rare cases death may occur from this disorder. Discuss the causes of death in Reiter's syndrome.

A. Massive necrosis of the submucosa and gastric ulceration may lead to diffuse gastrointestinal hemorrhage and this has been described as a cause of death in the early stages of the disease. In later stages, aortic valve insufficiency, heart block, and cardiovascular complications may result in a fatal event. Additionally, amyloidosis has been reported now on several occasions in chronic cases of Reiter's syndrome.

REF: Caughey, D. E. and Wakem, C. J., "A fatal case of Reiter's disease complicated by amyloidosis." Arth Rheum 16:5, 695-700, 1973.

196. Q. Although the distinction between ankylosing spondylitis and Reiter's syndrome may be difficult in some
cases, what are the usual distinguishing clinical features
that serve to separate these disorders?

A. In ankylosing spondylitis the onset is typically more
gradual than it is in Reiter's syndrome. Urethritis, conjunctivitis, skin and mucous membrane lesions are typical
of Reiter's syndrome, while in ankylosing spondylitis conjunctivitis, when it occurs, is unusual. Uveitis is perhaps
more commonly seen in ankylosing spondylitis than it is in
Reiter's syndrome. Peripheral joint involvement occurs in
90% of cases of Reiter's syndrome and in only 25% of ankylosing spondylitis. The hips and spine are frequently affected in ankylosing spondylitis. Hip involvement is unusual in Reiter's syndrome, although knee involvement is
extremely common. Sacroiliitis is more common in ankylosing spondylitis, and is usually symmetrical and bilateral.
When sacroiliitis occurs in Reiter's syndrome, it is more
apt to be unilateral and asymmetrical.

REF: Calin, A. "Reiter's syndrome," Med Clin North Am,
61:2, 365-376, 1977.

197. Q. Compare and contrast the spondyloarthritides
and rheumatoid arthritis in terms of their distribution,
prevalence, and historical perspective.

A. It has always been of interest that rheumatoid arthritis appears to be a relatively recent disorder. Whereas
data appear frequently to suggest that ankylosing spondylitis
and Reiter's syndrome were probably present as early as
3000 B.C., rheumatoid arthritis dates back to perhaps the
nineteenth century. The distribution of rheumatoid arthritis
is worldwide, although ankylosing spondylitis and Reiter's
syndrome have strong racial determinants. With the advent
of HLA tissue typing, it has now become clear that ankylosing spondylitis and Reiter's syndrome are far more frequent than was previously anticipated approaching the
incidence of rheumatoid arthritis.

REF: Calin, A. "Reiter's syndrome." Med Clin North Am,
61:2, 365-376, 1977.

198. Q. What is the typical "triad" of Reiter's syndrome?
Discuss the concept of "incomplete" Reiter's syndrome.

A. In 1916 Hans Reiter described the classical triad
of urethritis, conjunctivitis, and arthritis that now bears
his name. Thereafter, for many years the diagnosis was
made when all three elements of the triad were present.
However, not all three of these elements need be present
at any given moment, and they may be separated temporally.
With the discovery of tissue typing and the correlation of
the HLA-B27 antigen with Reiter's syndrome, the diagnosis
of incomplete Reiter's syndrome has now been made easier.
Hence, two or even one of the elements of the original classical triad may be present which may be enough for the diagnosis if other clinical and laboratory findings are present.

REF: Calin, A. "Reiter's syndrome." Med Clin North Am,
61:2, 365-376, 1977.

199. Q. What is the incidence of ocular involvement in
psoriatic arthritis?

A. Some type of ocular involvement may be seen in
up to 30% of patients with psoriatic arthritis. These types
of involvement include conjunctivitis, iritis, episcleritis,
and keratoconjunctivitis sicca. The presence of ocular involvement lends further support to the concept that psoriatic
arthritis has important links to the other spondyloarthritides
such as ankylosing spondylitis and Reiter's syndrome.

REF: Lambert, J.R. and Wright, V. "Eye inflammation in
psoriatic arthritis." Ann Rheum Dis 35, 354-356, 1976.

200. Q. What is the frequency of osteoarthritis in the elbows and shoulders of pneumatic drillers and what are therefore the implications to the concept that osteoarthritis is a "wear and tear" process of joints?

A. In a survey of 34 pneumatic drillers, osteoarthritis was noted in the elbows of only 2 subjects. Two others had generalized osteoarthritic changes, and 15 subjects were noted to have mild degenerative changes in the hands. The conclusion reached by the authors was that pneumatic drillers were not prone to develop osteoarthritis, casting doubt on the validity of osteoarthritis as a "wear and tear" disease.

REF: Burke, M.J., Fear, E.C., and Wright, V. "Bone and joint changes in pneumatic drillers." Ann Rheum Dis 36, 276-279, 1977.

201. Q. What would you expect to see in terms of osteoarthritic involvement of the knee and ankle in parachutists as compared to age-matched, less active subjects? Discuss.

A. Although degenerative osteoarthritis has always been considered a "wear and tear" arthritis, the frequency of osteoarthritic involvement of the knee or ankle in parachutists has been found to be comparable to that seen in less active age-matched individuals. This emphasizes the importance of factors other than trauma in the pathogenesis of osteoarthritis.

REF: Murray Leslie, C.F., Lintott, D.J., and Wright, V. "The knees and ankles in sport and veteran military parachutists." Ann Rheum Dis 36, 327-331, 1977.

202. Q. In professional atheletes and individuals very active in sports, what factors would tend to predispose these persons to the development of osteoarthritis?

A. It would appear that the most important factors statistically in the development of osteoarthritis are the presence of fractures through the joint line which almost inevitably lead to the subsequent development of osteoarthritis, and menisectomy of the knee which then increases the risk of developing degenerative joint disease in that joint.

REF: Murray Leslie, C.F., Lintott, D.J., and Wright, V. "The knee and ankles in sport and veteran military parachutists." Ann Rheum Dis 36, 327-331, 1977.

203. Q. What are the differences, if any, in parachutists and the subsequent development of degenerative discogenic and joint disease of the spine when compared to the development of osteoarthritis in the knees or ankles? Discuss.

A. In a study of veteran parachutists, there was no direct correlation between the development of intervertebral disc degeneration, spondylolysis or spondylolisthesis. This was true despite the rather frequent incidence of spinal trauma and fractures of the vertebrae, particularly T12. Therefore, it has been concluded that chronic trauma, such as parachuting, does not appear to predispose individuals to the development of degenerative joint disease either of the neck and spine, or of the ankles and knees.

REF: Murray Leslie, C.F., Lintott, D.J., and Wright, V. "The spine in sport and veteran military parachutists." Ann Rheum Dis 36, 332-342, 1977.

204. Q. In tasks that require repetitive stereotyped usage involving a power grip, what types of problems might one expect to see in the hands and wrists?

A. In general, the development of three types of industrially-related rheumatological problems have been associated with this type of work-related activity. These are (1) carpal tunnel syndrome, (2) tenosynovitis of the wrist with associated degenerative joint disease of the scapho-trapezoid joint, and (3) DeQuervain's tenosynovitis.

REF: Hadler, N.M., "Industrial rheumatology." Arth Rheum 20:4, 1019-1024, 1977.

205. Q. Discuss the development of low back pain in the context of an industrially related rheumatologic problem.

A. The development of low back pain is a frequent occurrence in workers engaged in a multitude of professions and occupations. In most studies, there has been a relationship between the frequency of low back pain and the requirement of repetitive lifting. However, degenerative joint disease on radiographs has not been correlated either with the type of task performed, the frequency of heavy lifting, or the degree of back pain. Clearly other factors are important in the pathogenesis of low back pain in the industrial setting.

REF: Hadler, N.M., "Industrial rheumatology." Arth Rheum 20:4, 1019-1024, 1977.

206. Q. What is meant by the term "industrial rheumatology" and what are the implications and projected goals for this emerging discipline?

A. There is little proof and virtually no reliable data that would suggest a significant relationship between repetitive industrial work patterns and the development of localized musculoskeletal rheumatological disorders. Aside from overt trauma and discrete fractures, the development of such chronic problems as degenerative osteoarthritis, calcific bursitis and tendinitis, discogenic cervical and lumbosacral disease, and other similar disorders does not appear to be significantly related to industrial work patterns. Although increased symptoms may appear due to this type of repetitive exertion, nonetheless there may not be any pathogenetic implications in this relationship which may be more provocative than causal. In the field of "industrial rheumatism" the tasks therefore are to better define these relationships by carefully and critically designing long term studies in an effort to determine which are the salient factors in the causation or exacerbation of these disorders.

REF: Hadler, N.M. "Industrial rheumatology." Arth Rheum 20:4, 1019-1024, 1977.

207. Q. What is intervertebral (osteo) chondrosis?

A. This is a relatively common condition in the elderly. Dehydration of the nucleus pulposus and degeneration is associated with flattening of the intervertebral disc and sclerosis of the adjacent vertebral bodies. Schmorl's nodes or

cartilaginous nodes are herniations of this disc material into the vertebral bodies above and below the affected disc
area.

REF: Resnick, D. "Disorders of the axial skeleton which
are lesser known, poorly recognized or misunderstood."
Bull Rheum Dis 28:2,3, 932-939, 1977-78.

208. Q. What is meant by spondylosis deformans?

A. This also is not an uncommon development in elderly patients. Disruption of Sharpey's fibers within the
anulus fibrosus of the intervertebral disc leads to disruption
and herniation of the disc. Elevation of the anterior long-
itudinal ligament and subsequent traction at that site results
in the characteristic radiographic findings of osteophyte
formation of variable size along the anterolateral aspect of
the vertebral column. The absence of disc space loss and
little if any bony sclerosis are characteristic.

REF: Resnick, D. "Disorders of the axial skeleton which
are lesser known, poorly recognized or misunderstood."
Bull Rheum Dis 28:2,3, 932-939, 1977-78.

209. Q. Discuss diffuse idiopathic skeletal hyperostosis.

A. This is a recently proposed term for ankylosing
hyperostosis or Forestier's syndrome. While originally
thought to be a process confined to the spine, it is now felt
to encompass both spinal and extra-spinal sites. Hence,
the term diffuse idiopathic skeletal hyperostosis has been
proposed to call attention to the fact that extra-spinal sites
are commonly seen.

REF: Resnick, D. "Disorders of the axial skeleton which
are lesser known, poorly recognized, or misunderstood."
Bull Rheum Dis 28:2,3, 932-939, 1977-78.

210. Q. What are the radiographic features of diffuse
idiopathic skeletal hyperostosis?

A. Radiographically, this entity is defined as follows:
(1) Flowing calcification and ossification of a "waxy" type
along the anterolateral aspect of no less than four contiguous

vertebral bodies. (2) Little adjacent bony sclerosis and relative preservation of the disc space. (3) Relative normalcy of the apophyseal joints and the sacroiliac joints.

REF: Resnick, D. "Disorders of the axial skeleton which are lesser known, poorly recognized or misunderstood." Bull Rheum Dis 28:2,3, 932-939, 1977-78.

211. Q. In osteoarthritis, what are the histological changes that are noted?

A. Initially the changes are focal, and with advanced disease they become more generalized. Cartilage destruction, fibrillation, cyst formation, sclerosis, and the appearance of marginal osteophytes are characteristic.

REF: Sweet, M.B.E., Thonar, J.M.A., Immelman, A.R., and Solomon, L. "Biochemical changes in progressive osteoarthritis." Ann Rheum Dis 36, 387-398, 1977.

212. Q. Describe the biochemistry of normal cartilage.

A. The macromolecular matrix of cartilage consists of a series of proteoglycans which lie in a meshwork of collagen. Chondroitin sulfate and keratin sulfate covalently linked to a protein core form the basis of the proteoglycan units. They possess a highly negative electrostatic charge which retards the progress of interstitial water.

REF: Sweet, M.B.E., Thonar, J.M.A., Immelman, A.R., and Solomon, L. "Biochemical changes in progressive osteoarthritis." Ann Rheum Dis 36, 387-398, 1977.

213. Q. What are the typical biochemical changes in osteoarthritic cartilage?

A. In the cartilage of osteoarthritis, the glycosaminoglycan content is markedly reduced, especially the keratin sulfate fraction. Chain length is reduced, and there is an increase in water content. Glycosaminoglycan aggregation

is reduced, and an increase in chondroitin 4 sulfate is
usually observed.

REF: Sweet, M.B.E., Thonar, J.M.A., Immelman, A.R.,
and Solomon, L. "Biochemical changes in progressive
osteoarthritis." Ann Rheum Dis 36, 387-398, 1977.

214. Q. Although the pathogenesis of osteoarthritis is not
yet known, comment on the current hypothetical model which
would best explain the existing biochemical evidence.

A. A large body of evidence suggests that the loss of
proteoglycan from osteoarthritic cartilage is probably due
to the effect of a variety of proteolytic enzymes released
during the destruction and fibrillation of cartilage. Loss of
proteoclycan is balanced by increased synthesis and both
appear to be proportional to the severity of the osteoarthritis. In later stages, the chondrocytes no longer are capable
of keeping up with the proteoglycan loss. As new cartilage
matrix is formed, biochemical changes include an increase
in chondroitin 4 sulfate and a decrease in keratin sulfate.

REF: Sweet, M.B.E., Thonar, J.M.A., Immelman, A.R.,
and Solomon, L. "Biochemical changes in progressive
osteoarthritis." Ann Rheum Dis 36, 387-398, 1977.

215. Q. Comment on the usefulness of the various nonsteroidal antiinflammatory drugs in osteoarthritis from a
conceptual point of view.

A. Osteoarthritis may well be a disease of metabolism of cartilage involving increased hydration together with
certain fundamental alterations in proteoglycans. In its
later stages, degenerative changes ensue and probably permanent changes occur which may then be irreversible. Although treatment with a variety of antiinflammatory drugs
has been in vogue for many years, there is some doubt that
these drugs are of any value in a disease which may be more
biochemical and degenerative as opposed to inflammatory by
its very nature. Long term use of these drugs may in fact
be harmful to the osteoarthritic process.

REF: Muir, H. "Molecular approach to the understanding
of osteoarthritis." Ann Rheum Dis 36, 199-208, 1977.

216. Q. In experimental joint homografts, describe the
results thus far obtained and comment on the mechanism
of rejection.

A. The results to date with joint homografting have
not been encouraging. Survival and function of joint homografts have varied from 4 weeks to 12 months. Synovial hypertrophy and inflammation are seen to occur following homografting with invasion of the donor by a "panus-like" synovitis
originating from remaining synovial tissue. Cartilage destruction is noted. This may be due to inflammatory or
immunological mechanisms.

REF: Yablon, I. G., Brandt., K. D. Delellis, R., and
Covall, D. "Destruction of joint homografts. An Experimental Study." Arth Rheum 20:8, 1526-1537, 1977.

217. Q. Describe the hip prosthesis first pioneered by Dr.
John Charnley as to its components.

A. The artificial hip joint is composed of two components. The acetabular component is made of plastic which
is a polyethylene substance. The femoral component is met-
allic and is generally inserted into the medullary cavity in
the proximal femur. Fixation of both components is by a
cement-like substance, methyl methacrylate.

REF: Harris, W. H. "Total hip replacement." New Engl J
Med 297:12, 650-651, 1977.

218. Q. Comment on the statistics that support the concept
of total hip replacement.

A. Approximately 75,000 such operations are performed yearly in the United States. Up to 90% of patients
followed for five years have a good to excellent result. In
a series reported by Charnley, his 10-year followup reveals
that only 20% of patients developed signs of looseness of the
femoral component or some type of failure of the procedure.

REF: Harris, W. H. "Total hip replacement." New Engl J
Med 297:12, 650-651, 1977.

219. Q. Describe the technique of cervical analgesic
discography.

A. The painful disc syndrome classically is the complex of pain associated with paresthesias involving the head,
shoulder, and upper arm, usually without demonstrable
neurologic deficits. Radiographs and cervical myelography
are generally relatively unremarkable other than for revealing degenerative changes. The injection of a local analgesic
agent into a disc suspected of being the responsible agent
for the painful complex will produce transient symptomatic
relief and full cervical mobility. Surgical fusion usually
will result in excellent postoperative results in patients so
evaluated and selected for surgery.

REF: Roth, D. A. "Cervical analgesic discography." JAMA
235:16, 1713-1714, 1976.

220. Q. Although chemical and enzymatic factors are considered of importance in the development of osteoarthritis,
mechanical aspects are similarly of significance. Discuss.

A. In general, the initial triggering event in the development of degenerative joint disease would appear to be
some type of increased stress on the cartilage. This may
be obvious, such as in joint incongruity, or it may be subtle.
Bony changes occur early in the osteoarthritic process and
frequently help determine the extent of cartilaginous damage.
The type of stress that appears to be most undesirable from
a mechanical point of view is that of repetitive impulsive
loading. This often leads to tensile fatigue of the soft tissues, subchondral bone trabecular microfractures, increased
bone stiffness as healing occurs, and cartilage degeneration.

REF: Radin, E. L. "Mechanical aspects of osteoarthritis."
Bull Rheum Dis 26:7, 862-865, 1975-76.

221. Q. What is chondromalacia and how does it differ
from osteoarthritis in the early stages?

A. Chondromalacia, or "softening of the cartilage,"
is in reality a nonprogressive fibrillation of cartilage. A
frequent site for this process is in the patella. It differs from

the early cartilaginous changes seen in degenerative joint disease by the absence of subchondral bone changes such as trabecular disruption and microfractures.

REF: Radin, E. L. "Mechanical aspects of osteoarthritis." Bull Rheum Dis 26:7, 862-865, 1975-76.

222. Q. Clearly great advances have occurred in the field of orthopedic surgery and prosthetic replacement of severely osteoarthritic joints. Although the advances in the field of biochemical and enzymatic understanding of osteoarthritis are still preliminary, many research physicians are hopeful that it may one day be possible to restore an osteoarthritic joint by biochemical means. Comment on the directions this type of research has taken in the recent literature.

A. It has now become evident that articular cartilage is not an inert material, but instead is a highly complex and vigorous biochemical and enzymatic matrix. Thus, it is fully capable of highly reparative reaction under appropriate circumstances. Theoretically, it should be possible to restore degenerated cartilage by either increasing the process of repair, or alternatively by decreasing the enzymatic destruction of the cartilage. In this context, recent research has indicated that uridine diphosphate can increase proteoglycan synthesis in the articular cartilage of the rabbit both in vivo and in vitro. Salicylates have been shown to inhibit the degeneration of cartilage under certain circumstances. Therefore, the hope that someday a biochemical cure for osteoarthritis will be developed is not an altogether unrealistic notion.

REF: Mankin, H. J. "The reaction of articular cartilage to injury and osteoarthritis." New Engl J Med 291:24, 25, 1285-1340, 1974.

223. Q. As a consultant for a large factory employing many laborers, what type of considerations would be pertinent in attempting to reduce the incidence of low back pain in the laborers of that factory.

A. Low back pain is a frequent health and economic problem for a large segment of the working population. Of importance are prolonged periods of standing or sitting, which seem to increase the incidence of low back pain considerably. On the other hand, those workers who are able to interrupt their work by sitting or standing for brief periods suffer far less low back pain. Although pre-employment radiographic examination of the low back did not appear to reliably predict low back pain and injuries, nonetheless, decreased time lost from work was noted by allowing better placement of workers to jobs.

REF: Magora, A. "Investigation of the relation between low back pain and occupation. 3 physical requirements: sitting, standing and weight lifting." Industr Med Surg 41, 5-9, 1972.

Moreton, R. D. , "The role of preplacement roentgenogram examination of the spine in evaluation of low back pain." South Med J 67, 1105-1110, 1974.

224. Q. Describe the usual psychological profile found by psychometric testing in patients with low back pain.

A. In general, these patients have been found to possess the following psychological characteristics: latent depression, tendency toward invalidism, repeated conflict and challenges to the physicians caring for the patient to find the correct diagnosis for the back pain. Treatment with antidepressant medication and sleeping pills appeared to improve symptoms in some of these patients.

REF: Forrest, A. J. , and Wolking, S. N. "Marked depression in men with low back pain." Rheumatol Rehab 13, 148-153, 1974.

Sternback, R. A. , Murphy, R. W. , Akeson, W. H. , et. al. "Chronic low back pain: the "low back loser." Postgrad Med 53, 135-138, 1973.

225. Q. Describe the initial results with chymopapain injections for discogenic disease. What is the status of this procedure in the United States at this time?

A. Approximately two thirds of patients given intradiscal injections of this enzyme appeared to respond nicely. However, although the procedure is used in Canada and other countries, its use in the United States has been curtailed by the Food and Drug Administration when it denied Phase IV investigations with this drug.

REF: Graham, C. E. "Backache and sciatica: a report of 90 patients treated by intradiscal injection of chymopapain (Disease)." Med J Aust 1, 5-8, 1974.

226. Q. Discuss the complications of total hip replacement.

A. Thromboembolic complications are probably the most commonly noted, and when patients are not given adequate anticoagulant prophylaxis, this problem has approached the 50% level. Sepsis is now seen in about 1% of cases, and frequently this is a late occurrence months or even years after the surgery. Other complications include dislocation, heterotopic ossification, failure of the osteotomized trochanter to heal, fracture of the femur, palsy of the sciatic or femoral nerve, loosening of the femoral component, and fracture of the metal stem of the femoral component.

REF: Harris W. H. "Total hip replacement." New Engl J Med 297:12, 650-651, 1977.

227. Q. Comment on the total knee replacement technique.

A. The knee is a much more difficult joint to replace surgically. Many designs of components are available attesting to the fact that no uniformly successful prosthesis is available as of this time. Hinged prostheses appear to be the most problematical. Failure rates of 15 to 25% in the first several years following surgery are not uncommon. It is advisable to defer total knee replacement, particularly in the younger patient, until such a time as further experience and data are available. There is some evidence that the newer designs may have improved function and survival data.

REF: Harris, W. H. "Total hip replacement." New Engl J Med 297:12, 650-651, 1977.

XI. GOUT AND PSEUDOGOUT

228. Q. Discuss the preliminary criteria for the classification of acute gout.

A. In a study of over 700 patients with gout, pseudogout,
and other rheumatic disorders, the following diagnostic criteria emerged in an effort to define and clarify the diagnosis
of gout. (1) Typical urate crystals in the joint fluid, (2) soft
tissue urate deposits in the form of a tophus, demonstrated
either by chemical determination or polarized light, and in
the absence of these definitive parameters, the presence of
certain clinical laboratory and radiographic phenomena as
listed below. Six of twelve of these parameters would serve
to confirm the diagnosis: (a) inflammation restricted to one
day, (b) multiple attacks, (c) monoarticular arthritis, (d) red-
ness, (e) involvement of the MTP joint of the great toe,
(f) unilateral great toe MTP involvement, (g) unilateral tarsal involvement, (h) suspected tophus, (i) hyperuricemia,
(j) asymmetric swelling, (k) cystic lesions without erosions
in the subcortical bone, (l) negative cultures.

REF: Wallace, S. L., Robinson, H., Masi, A. T., et. al.
"Preliminary criteria for the classification of the acute
arthritis of primary gout." Arth Rheum 20:3, 895-900,
1977.

229. Q. In gout, describe the usual radiographic changes
that may be seen.

A. Perhaps the most characteristic radiographic sign
is the "overhanging edge" described by Martel in gout. However, other changes include cortical erosions of bone in the
subchondral region and at avascular sites of ligamentous
and tendinous insertions, sclerotic margins and lack of
osteoporosis or joint space narrowing.

REF: Trentham, D. E., and Masi, A. T. "Chronic synovitis
in gout simulating rheumatoid arthritis." JAMA 235:13,
1358-1360, 1976.

230. Q. Comment on gout and chronic synovitis simulating rheumatoid arthritis.

A. Gout and rheumatoid arthritis have traditionally been thought of as being mutually exclusive. However, in certain instances, gout may mimic rheumatoid arthritis clinically and radiographically, emphasizing the need for critical differential diagnosis. Involvement of the knees and wrists may simulate rheumatoid disease both from a clinical as well as from a radiographic perspective. Chronic synovial inflammation, thus, may be a feature of gout.

REF: Trentham, D. E. and Masi, A. T. "Chronic synovitis in gout simulating rheumatoid arthritis." JAMA 235:13, 1358-1360, 1976.

231. Q. Discuss the current concepts of the pathogenesis of podagra in gout.

A. Urate solubility determines whether or not uric acid crystals will precipitate from a synovial effusion. In general, there appears to be some correlation between an acute attack of gout and previous trauma, injury, or degenerative osteoarthritis in the MTP joint. It has been hypothesized that the mechanism by which acute podagra develops in the MTP joint is by the prior induction of a localized articular effusion in the MTP joint either by injury or by degenerative changes. Because water leaves a joint effusion far more rapidly than urate, the concentration of uric acid will rise during the night as water leaves the joint space. When the critical solubility of urate is reached, uric acid crystals precipitate, inducing acute podagra.

REF: Simkin, P. A. "The pathogenesis of podagra." Ann Intern Med 86, 230-233, 1977.

232. Q. How significant is hyperuricemia in relationship to clinical gout in population studies such as the Framingham study?

A. In population studies of which perhaps the classic study is that of the Framingham survey, it has become clear that rather modest levels of hyperuricemia are the rule in gouty patients. Perhaps 38% of gouty subjects have serum uric acid levels in the normal range, while another 39% have serum uric acid levels below 8.0 mgm per dl.

REF: Hall, A.P., Barry, P.E. and Dawber, T.R., et.al. "Epidemiology of gout and hyperuricemia. A long term population study." Am J Med 42, 27-37, 1967.

233. Q. The big toe has been the classical site of gouty involvement. How often does involvement of the great toe occur in gout?

A. It has been estimated that at least 60% of patients will present with podagra initially, while another 40% will eventually develop involvement with further observation of the clinical course.

REF: Simkin, P.A. "The pathogenesis of podagra." Ann Intern Med 86, 230-233, 1977.

234. Q. Discuss the causes of secondary hyperuricemia that are most commonly seen in the clinical context.

A. Chronic myeloproliferative diseases, lympho-proliferative diseases, and the treatment of these disorders with cytotoxic drugs, psoriasis, renal failure, starvation, obesity, and the use of certain drugs such as low dose salicylates, alcohol, diuretics, and pyrazinamide are all associated with hyperuricemia. Diabetic acidosis, glycogen storage disease of the type I variety, sarcoidosis, hyperparathyroidism, lead poisoning, and Down's syndrome are additional causes.

REF: Klinenberg, J.R., Bluestone, R., Schlosstein, L., et.al. "Urate deposition disease." Ann Intern Med 78, 99-111, 1973.

235. Q. Discuss the significance of urate binding to plasma proteins.

A. Because only an estimated 25% of patients with concentrations of uric acid exceeding solubility limits develop clinical gout, it is obvious that other factors are of importance to the development of uric acid precipitation. Therefore, it has been proposed that urate binding to plasma proteins may be a significant factor. Urate is avidly bound to albumin, and this binding influences not only urate deposition, but also the renal excretion of uric acid. Many of the well known uricosuric drugs themselves interfere with urate binding, such as salicylates, phenylbutazone, sulfinpyrazone, indomethacin, and probenecid.

REF: Klinenberg, J.R., Bluestone, R., Schlosstein, L., et. al. "Urate deposition disease." Ann Intern Med 78, 99-111, 1973.

236. Q. Discuss the relationship of serum uric acid levels to the frequency of clinical gout and uric acid nephrolithiasis.

A. The serum uric acid level is directly correlated with acute gout and kidney stone formation. In the Framingham study, men with uric acid levels consistently below 6 mgm per cent developed gout very rarely, probably less than 1%. As the serum uric acid level increased to 9 mgm per cent or greater, more than 90% of subjects developed gout. Stone formation was seen in 12.7% of men with uric acid levels of 7.0 mgm percent or more, and in 40% with levels of 9.0 mgm per cent or greater.

REF: Healy, L.A. and Hall, A.P. "The epidemiology of hyperuricemia." Bull Rheum Dis 20:8, 600-603, 1970.

237. Q. Discuss the renal tubular transport of uric acid with the relative contributions from the glomerulus, proximal and distal tubule, and collecting ducts.

A. Filtration of uric acid occurs at the glomerulus and accounts for virtually complete filtration from the blood. In the proximal tubule, 98% of the filtrate is then reabsorbed. Further along in the proximal tubule, perhaps 50% or so is then secreted, which then again is reabsorbed in the proximal tubule and the loop of Henle. Finally, it has been estimated that the final excretion of urate is on the order of 10% of the original amount filtered at the glomerulus.

REF: Diamond, H.S., Meisel, A., and Kaplan, D. "Renal tubular transport of urate in man." Bull Rheum Dis, 27:1, 876-881, 1976-77.

238. Q. What is the mechanism of hyperuricemia in renal failure?

A. The excretion of uric acid is relatively well preserved in renal failure as the number of functioning nephron units declines. However, as renal failure advances, the number of functioning nephrons falls, and the clearance of urate diminishes. This is despite the fact that the actual excretion of urate per individual nephron increases. In mild renal failure, there is decreased reabsorption of secreted urate at the tubular level. In advanced renal disease, the amount of reabsorbed urate decreases as to both filtered and secreted urate.

REF: Diamond, H.S., Meisel, A., and Kaplan, D. "Renal tubular transport of urate in man." Bull Rheum Dis, 27:1 876-881, 1976-77.

239. Q. In gouty subjects, what is the relative urate clearance ratio as compared to normal subjects?

A. For a given serum uric acid level, the urate clearance will be somewhat diminished when compared to normal subjects. The cause is not known, although it may be in part related to disorders of tubular handling of urate.

REF: Diamond, H.S., Meisel, A., and Kaplan, D. "Renal tubular transport of urate in man." Bull Rheum Dis, 27:1, 876-881, 1976-77.

240. Q. What are the basic mechanisms of hyperuricemia in man, and comment as to their relative frequencies?

A. Hyperuricemia, conceptually, may result from either (1) urate production, which accounts for perhaps 25% of patients, (2) decreased excretion, accounting for another 25%, or (3) a combination of the two (50%).

REF: Holmes, E.W., Kelley, W.N., and Wyngaarden, J.B. "Control of purine biosynthesis in normal and pathologic states." Bull Rheum Dis 26:4, 848-853, 1975-76.

241. Q. On an enzymatic level, discuss three mechanisms by which there may be an increase in de novo synthesis of uric acid.

A. Enzymatic alterations leading to increased de novo overproduction of purines may be categorized into three major groupings. (1) Increased availability of PP-ribose-P. (2) Decreased intracellular pool of purine ribonucleotides. (3) Increased glutamine concentration.

REF: Holmes, E.W., Kelley, W.N., and Wyngaarden, J.B. "Control of purine biosynthesis in normal and pathologic states." Bull Rheum Dis 26:4, 848 - 853, 1975-76.

242. Q. Discuss the mechanism of hyperuricemia in HGPRT deficiency.

A. Hypoxanthine guanine phosphoribosyl transferase (HGPRT) deficiency results in an accumulation of PP-ribose-P which is one of its substrates. As PP-ribose-P increases, it leads to greater generation of IMP, inosine, hypoxanthine, xanthine, and finally uric acid.

REF: Holmes, E.W., Kelley, W.N., and Wyngaarden, J.B. "Control of purine biosynthesis in normal and pathologic states." Bull Rheum Dis 26:4, 848-853, 1975-76.

243. Q. What are the features of the Lesch-Nyhan syndrome?

A. The Lesch-Nyhan syndrome refers to a virtually complete deficiency of the HGPRT enzyme, which is a sex-linked trait. Therefore, it occurs in males and presents with hyperuricemia, hyperuricaciduria, uric acid renal stones, self-multilating compulsive neurological disorder, choreoathetosis, spasticity, and mental retardation.

REF: Holmes, E.W., Kelley, W.N., and Wyngaarden, J.B. "Control of purine biosynthesis in normal and pathologic states." Bull Rheum Dis 26:4, 848-853, 1976-76.

244. Q. Describe the typical findings in an individual with a partial HGPRT deficiency.

A. In these individuals, the neurological signs and symptoms are either nonexistent or very mild. However,

gouty arthritis and urinary renal calculi may occur at an
early age. Hyperuricemia and hyperuricaciduria are
present.

REF: Holmes, E. W. , Kelley, W. N. , and Wyngaarden,
J. B. "Control of purine biosynthesis in normal and pathologic states." Bull Rheum Dis 26:4, 848-853, 1975-76.

245. Q. What are the indications for allopurinol in the
treatment of hyperuricemia?

    A. Because allopurinol is a somewhat more toxic
agent than probenecid, the latter is probably preferable
in the usual case of hyperuricemia unless any of the following factors are present: (1) Urinary uric acid greater than
900 mgm per 24 hours, (2) Documented overproduction of
uric acid, (3) Anticipated acute hyperuricemia such as with
cytotoxic drug therapy, (4) Renal failure with a creatinine
clearance less than 40 cc per minute, (5) Uric acid calculi,
and (6) Evidence that other uricosuric agents are either
ineffective or poorly tolerated.

REF: Steele, T. H. "Hyperuricemia and the kidney." The
Kidney, 8:2, 7-10, 1975.

246. Q. Discuss the use of prophylactic colchicine in the
therapy of intercritical gout as to its usefulness and toxicity.

    A. The use of colchicine as a prophylactic measure
in intercritical gout has been shown to reduce the number
of attacks from an average of 6 attacks per year to 2. 3
attacks, in one study. Side effects such as nausea, diarrhea, abdominal pain, and transaminase elevation were not
infrequent, however. The authors concluded that although
this use of colchicine appeared effective, it did not eliminate
attacks, and unpleasant side effects were not uncommon.

REF: Paulus, H. E. , Schlosstein, H. , Godfrey, R. G. ,
et. al. "Prophylactic colchicine therapy of intercritical
gout." Arth Rheum 15:5, 609-614, 1974.

247. Q. Discuss the proposed mechanisms that result in the appearance of uric acid crystals in the synovial fluid.

A. Two mechanisms have been proposed to account for the appearance of free urate crystals within synovial fluid. (1) Enzymatic degradation of proteoglycans from cartilage may result in the "unloading" of urate into the synovial fluid, and (2) decreased $alpha_1$ and $alpha_2$ urate binding globulins would then lead to an increase in free urate leading to increased crystalization.

REF: Spilberg, I. "Current concepts of the mechanisms of acute inflammation in gouty arthritis." Arth Rheum 18:2, 129-134, 1975.

248. Q. Discuss a mechanism by which an acute gouty attack would follow the institution of allopurinol in a patient with hyperuricemia.

A. Allopurinol is a xanthine oxidase inhibitor which when given to a patient with hyperuricemia may produce a sudden fall in serum uric acid levels. As the concentration of uric acid falls in body fluids, irregular dissolution of the surface deposits of uric acid in joints would lead to release of undissolved crystals, thereby precipitating acute clinical gouty arthritis.

REF: Spilberg, I. "Current concepts of the mechanism of acute inflammation in gouty arthritis." Arth Rheum 18:2, 129-134, 1975.

249. Q. An intriguing problem in gout has always been what factor or factors may be responsible for the eventual termination of an acute gouty attack. Discuss the proposed mechanisms.

A. The events which lead to a spontaneous termination of an acute gouty attack have not been elucidated although several factors are felt to be of importance. (1) Increased blood flow and diffusion out of the joint cavity facilitates removal of free urate, (2) lysosomal myeloperoxidase is capable of breaking down urate to allantoin, and

(3) as a response to stress, increased adrenal corticosteroids may act as antiinflammatory agents in suppressing an acute attack.

REF: Spilberg, I. "Current concepts of the mechanism of acute inflammation in gouty arthritis." Arth Rheum 18:2, 129-134, 1975.

250. Q. Describe the sequence of events felt to occur in crystal-induced arthritis.

A. Perhaps the only critical requirements in crystal-induced arthritis are crystals and polymorphonuclear leukocytes. Phagocytosis of crystals results in rupture of lysosomal membranes and release of chemotactic factors attracting other polymorphonuclear cells. This amplification process leads to a high concentration of lysosomal products and proteases inside the joint cavity. These proteases result in soft tissue injury and cartilage destruction. Kinins may play a role in the inflammatory process, particularly later in the course of the arthritis.

REF: Spilberg, I. "Current concepts of the mechanism of acute inflammation in gouty arthritis." Arth Rheum 18:2, 129-134, 1975.

251. Q. Discuss the various patterns that may be seen clinically in calcium pyrophosphate dihydrate crystal deposition disease.

A. The classical presentation of calcium pyrophosphate crystal deposition disease is that of "pseudogout." The term is derived from gout and suggests a close similarity between gout and pseudogout in clinical symptoms. However, variants of the CPPD syndrome include a "rheumatoid" pattern, an "osteoarthritis" pattern, an asymptomatic (lanthantic) pattern, and a "pseudoneurotrophic" pattern.

REF: McCarty, D.J. "Diagnostic mimicry in arthritis: Patterns of joint involvement associated with calcium pyrophosphate dihydrate crystal deposits." Bull Rheum Dis 25:5, 804-809, 1974-75.

252. Q. Discuss the possibility that calcium pyrophosphate crystal deposition disease may mimic ankylosing spondylitis.

A. Stiffening and straightening of the lumbar spine has been described in calcium pyrophosphate deposition disease in familial cases both from Czechoslovakia and Chile. Actual bony ankylosis may be seen, making the differential diagnosis difficult. The HLA-B27 antigen, however, helps to separate these unusual cases.

REF: McCarty, D.J. "Diagnostic mimicry in arthritis: Patterns of joint involvement associated with calcium pyrophosphate dihydrate crystal deposits." Bull Rheum Dis 25:5, 804-809, 1974-75.

253. Q. What factors influence the clinical expression of calcium pyrophosphate deposition disease from a "pseudogout" presentation to patterns resembling rheumatoid arthritis and osteoarthritis?

A. Calcium pyrophosphate deposition disease is found in association with chondrocalcinosis which appears to be associated with cartilaginous degeneration. These observations would account for the pattern of "osteoarthritis" that may be seen. The polyarticular distribution of CPPD may lead to a "rheumatoid" presentation. Finally, crystal-induced inflammation is a dose-related phenomenon accounting for the many patterns of intensity which may be seen from the "pseudogout" attack to the subclinical form.

REF: McCarty, D.J. "Diagnostic mimicry in arthritis: Patterns of joint involvement associated with calcium pyrophosphate dihydrate crystal deposits." Bull Rheum Dis 25:5, 804-809, 1975-75.

254. Q. Discuss the association of hyperparathyroidism, chondrocalcinosis, and pseudogout and comment on the effect of parathyroidectomy.

A. Hyperparathyroidism is well known to be associated with both chondrocalcinosis and pseudogout (calcium pyrophosphate dihydrate crystal synovitis). The frequency with which chondrocalcinosis is seen in hyperparathyroidism has been estimated at 18% to 24%. When parathyroidectomy was performed in patients with hyperparathyroidism and pseudogout, no significant effect was noted on the attacks of pseudogout or on the chondrocalcinosis as noted radiographically.

REF: Pritchard, M. H. and Jessop, J. D. "Chondrocalcinosis in primary hyperparathyroidism." Ann Rheum Dis 36, 141-151, 1977.

255. Q. Comment on the relationship between calcium pyrophosphate crystal deposition disease and parathyroid hormone levels.

A. In patients with chondrocalcinosis, there appears to be an association between elevated parathormone levels. This further extends the association between chondrocalcinosis, pseudogout, and hyperparathyroidism, although the relationships are as yet unclear.

REF: Phelps, P. and Hawker, C. D. "Serum parathyroid hormone levels in patients with calcium pyrophosphate crystal deposition disease (chondrocalcinosis, pseudogout)." Arth Rheum 16.5, 590-596, 1973.

256. Q. What is the significance of fine linear calcifications in the Achilles or quadriceps tendons as might be seen on conventional radiographs?

A. In a series of patients with chondrocalcinosis, the Achilles and quadriceps tendons were noted to contain fine linear calcifications. This finding could be of potential importance in suggesting the presence of disease.

REF: Gerster, J. C. , Baud, C. A. , Lagier, R. , et. al. "Tendon calcifications in chondrocalcinosis." Arth Rheum 20:2, 717-722, 1977.

257. Q. Compare and contrast gout and pseudogout in the clinical context.

A. Gout is predominantly a disease of men while pseudogout occurs in both men and women nearly to an equal degree. The small joints are affected in gout, notably the great toe. Larger joints are frequently affected in pseudogout, especially the knee. Although both gout and pseudogout may resemble one another precisely as to the type of inflammation seen, the attacks in pseudogout tend to be somewhat milder and appear to increase in severity at a slower rate. The uric acid is regularly elevated in gout, but may also be elevated in pseudogout in perhaps 20% of patients. The response to colchicine may be seen in both disorders, although improvement is more nearly the rule in gout.

REF: Boyle, J.A. and Buchanan, W.W. "Clinical Rheumatology," Blackwell Scientific Publications, Oxford and Edingburgh, 1971, p. 219-261.

258. Q. Describe the type of crystals seen in gout and pseudogout and how the diagnosis should best be made.

A. The most precise method of determining whether a crystal is a monosodium urate crystal or a calcium pyrophosphate dihydrate crystal is to employ the technique of color compensated polarized light microscopy. The uric acid crystal when so viewed will be negatively birefringent, while the calcium pyrophosphate crystal will be positively birefringent. Under plain polarized light, architectural differences between these crystals may be used to make the differentiation. Uric acid crystals are typically "needle" shaped, while calcium pyrophosphate crystals tend to be somewhat more "rhomboid" in appearance.

REF: Fagan, T.J. and Lidsky, M.D. "Compensated polarized light microscopy using cellophane adhesive tape." Arth Rheum 17:3, 256-262, 1974.

259. Q. Discuss the proposed pathogenetic mechanisms in the development of gouty nephropathy.

A. Three basic mechanisms have been proposed. (1) A "blockade" by uric acid within the kidney tubules may lead to acute oliguric renal failure. (2) Chronic interstitial nephritis may be due to migration of intratubular uric acid crystals into the renal interstitium where they produce an inflammatory response. (3) Uric acid calculi lead to obstructive and infectious complications further adding to the renal disease.

REF: Bluestone, R., Waisman, J., and Klinenberg, J.R. "The gouty kidney." Semin Arth Rheum 7:2, 97-113, 1977.

260. Q. In the hyperuricemic patient, what further clinical variables would you expect to be correlated with the serum uric acid level, and which of these seem to be the most important and independent variables?

A. The variables that have been associated with hyperuricemia include renal disease, weight, blood pressure, hypercholesterolemia, hypertriglyceridemia, diabetes mellitus, and atherosclerosis. In a regression analysis of multiple variables, it was found that nonadipose, lean body weight and serum creatinine levels appeared to be perhaps the most important determinants of serum uric acid. The authors concluded that for practical purposes, the patient with hyperuricemia should be considered to be at higher risk to develop coronary artery disease and diabetes mellitus.

REF: Fessel, W. J. and Barr, G. D. "Uric acid, lean body weight, and creatinine interactions: Results from regression analysis of 78 variables." Semin Arth Rheum 7:2, 115-121, 1977.

261. Q. List the various lymphokines produced by lymphocytes which are known to be biologically active.

A. The list of substances known to be biologically
active released by lymphocytes is one which is growing with
newly identified compounds. A partial list of the more prominent lymphokines is as follows: macrophage inhibitory factor (MIF), macrophage activating factor, chemotactic factor, skin nuclear cells, lymphocytotoxins, growth inhibitory
factor, skin reactive factor, blastogenic factor, interferon,
and transfer factor.

REF: David, J.R. "Lymphocyte mediators and cellular
hypersensitivity." New Engl J Med 288:3, 143-149, 1973.

262. Q. Discuss the composition of peripheral blood lymphocytes as well as thoracic duct lymphocytes, their location
in the lymph nodes and spleen.

A. In the peripheral blood T-lymphocytes account
for 60 to 80% while B-cells number 20 to 30%. The thoracic duct is almost entirely composed of T-cells (85 to 90%)
as compared to B-cells (10 to 15%). In the lymph node,
T-cells are generally in the paracortical region, whereas
B-cells are located principally in the germinal centers,
subcapsular area, and in the medullary cords. In the spleen,
T-cells are in a periarteriolar location, while B-cells are
in germinol centers and in the red pulp.

REF: Winkelstein, A. and Rabin, B.S. "Lymphocyte biology. Part One." Bull Rheum Dis 25:7, 816-821, 1974-75.

263. Q. Discuss the presumed biological functions and
significance of humoral immunity (B-cells) and cellular
immunity (T-cells).

A. Humoral immunity deals primarily with contain-
ment and encapsulation of pyogenic bacteria such as the pneu-
mococci, streptococci, and so forth. In transplantation
rejection reactions, humoral immunity is responsible for
the "hyperacute" rejection. In terms of tumor immunity, a

role for immunologic enhancement has been proposed. In diseases of autoimmunity, pathogenic immune complexes may be formed which are then capable of renal disease such as in systemic lupus erythematosus. Cellular immunity deals with intracellular organisms which includes many bacteria such as the tubercle bacillus, viruses, protozoa, and fungi. It represents the major mechanism of transplantation rejection. In tumor immunity, the elimination of tumor cells is of prime importance. Finally, certain autoimmune disorders such as Hashimoto's thyroiditis appear to be related to T-cells and cell mediated immunity.

REF: Winkelstein, A. and Rabin, B.S. "Lymphocyte biology. Part One." Bull Rheum Dis 25:7, 816-821, 1974-75.

264. Q. Characterize T-cells and B-cells by laboratory techniques that are presently available.

A. Morphologically, lymphocytes appear rather similar, and it is not possible to differentiate T-cells from B-cells other than by certain immunobiological properties. As a rule, T-cells do not contain surface immunoglobulin or complement receptors and similarly do not carry a receptor for the Fc-fragment. However, E-rosettes form readily with sheep erythrocytes. Stimulation with a variety of mitogens may be demonstrated, including phytohemagglutinin, concanavalin-A, homologous lymphocytes, and pokeweed. In contrast to T-cells, B-cells carry receptors for immunoglobulins, complement, and the Fc-fragment, and do not form rosettes with sheep erythrocytes. A response to pokeweed may be elicited, but other mitogens do not appear to produce very significant stimulation.

REF: Winkelstein, A. and Rabin, B.S. "Lymphocyte biology. Part Two." Bull Rheum Dis 25:8, 822-827, 1974-75.

265. Q. As a physician who would be interested in obtaining an assessment of T-cell function in your patient, discuss the presently available laboratory techniques for doing this.

A. The following techniques are used to evaluate T-cell function. (1) Peripheral blood lymphocyte counts and histological examination of lymph nodes for thymic dependent areas. (2) Skin test reactivity and DNCB sensitization.

(3) Response in vitro to mitogens.   (4) Evaluation of T-cells by E-rosettes.   (5) Measurement of lymphokine generation and release.

REF: Winkelstein, A., and Rabin, B. S. "Lymphocyte biology. Part Two." Bull Rheum Dis 25:8, 822-827, 1974-75.

266. Q. What techniques are available to you as a physician to assess B-cell function ?

A.   (1) Quantitative immunoglobulin determinations, serum protein electrophoresis and immunoelectrophoresis. (2) Measurement of naturally occurring anti-A or anti-B red cell agglutinins and response to various primary and secondary antigens such as measles, influenza, and so on.   (3) B-cell enumeration by the techniques of immunofluorescence using anti-immunoglobulin or rosette formation with sheep erythrocytes coated with complement.   (4) Lymph node biopsy with histologic examination of thymic independent areas and the number of plasma cells in the bone marrow. (5) Stimulation with pokeweed mitogen.

REF: Winkelstein, A. and Rabin, B. S. "Lymphocyte biology. Part Two." Bull Rheum Dis 25:8, 822-827, 1974-75.

267. Q. Discuss the results of lymphocyte stimulation with hepatitis-B surface antigen in patients with acute and chronic hepatitis-B infections and comment on their significance.

A.   In acute hepatitis-B infections, cell mediated responses were absent during the acute phase of the infection, but reappeared and remained normal during convalescence and for up to six years thereafter. In type-B chronic hepatitis, patients with active disease and persistent transaminase elevation appeared to have reduced reactivity with hepatitis-B surface antigen.

REF: Tong, M. J., Wallace, A. M., Peters, R. L., and Reynolds, T. B. "Lymphocyte stimulation in hepatitis-B infections." New Engl J Med 293:7, 318-322, 1975.

268. Q. What is meant by the "T-cell lymphomas" and comment on the significance of the T-lymphocyte in these disorders.

A. The term "T-cell lymphomas" has been proposed for mycosis fungoides, the Sezary syndrome, and related cutaneous lymphomas such as lymphomatoid papulosis, and so forth. These neoplastic diseases appear to be composed primarily of T-cells which are probably monoclonal. The anergy so frequently a feature of these diseases is due to reduced numbers of normal T-cells.

REF: Lutzner, M., Edelson, R., Schein, P., et.al. "Cutaneous T-cell lymphomas: The Sezary syndrome, mycosis, fungoides, and related disorders." Ann Intern Med 83:534-552, 1975.

269. Q. What is the effect of therapeutic and physiologic doses of aspirin on lymphocyte transformation as measured by phytohemagglutinin and mixed lymphocyte culture techniques?

A. Initial reports in the literature suggested that aspirin was capable of producing lymphocyte suppression, and the issue of aspirin producing an effect on delayed hypersensitivity was raised as a possible mechanism of action. However, more recent data discredit a significant effect on lymphocyte function as measured by conventional techniques including response to phytohemagglutinin and mixed lymphocyte culture techniques.

REF: Smith, M.J., Hotch, M., and Davis, K. "Aspirin and lymphocyte transformation." Ann Intern Med 83:509-511, 1975.

270. Q. Comment on the data regarding T-cells and B-cells in rheumatoid arthritis, and the significance and reliability of such data.

A. Measurements of B-cells in rheumatoid arthritis has been primarily accomplished by measuring Ig and complement receptors. Measurement of T-cells has been by sheep cell rosette formation and by antithymocyte serum. In general, the results from one laboratory to another have differed widely. This may be because these techniques have not yet become sufficiently standardized to allow for comparative interpretation. Some studies suggest that there may be an increase in B-cells, while others suggest that there is a decrease, and still other studies show no significant changes. Similar data have been obtained with T-cell enumeration attempts. Certainly, it is clear that more work needs to be done in this important area.

REF: Messner, R. P. "Clinical aspects of T- and B-lymphocytes in rheumatic diseases." Arth Rheum 17:4, 339-346, 1974.

271. Q. Discuss the factors of importance in how lymphocytes appear to kill tumor cells.

A. Lymphocytes initially begin the process of killing tumor cells by active movement enabling the plasma membranes of the lymphocyte and the tumor cells to come into direct contact. The second stage is the establishment of a firm adhesion between these plasma membranes, a process which is facilitated by magnesium but also to a lesser extent by calcium ions. The third stage involves a prolonged contact between the plasma membranes of the lymphocyte and the tumor cell in the presence of calcium ions. The final stage of tumor cell lysis occurs as a result of increased tumor cell membrane permeability and increased osmotic intracellular pressures within the tumor cell. Lymphocytic membrane proteases appear to be instrumental in this process, which can continue without the further involvement of either the lymphocyte or the calcium or magnesium ions.

REF: Allison, A. C. and Ferluga, J. "How lymphocytes kill tumor cells." New Engl J Med 295:3, 165-167, 1976.

272. Q. Discuss the current theoretical notions of autoimmunity in terms of pathogenesis.

A. Certainly there is no clear idea of the pathogenetic mechanisms in the various autoimmune disorders such as systemic lupus erythematosus, rheumatoid arthritis, and similar disorders. However, several important factors have emerged from ongoing research in this area. Genetic predisposition undoubtedly is a factor of major importance, although by itself it does not appear to be sufficient for the development of these disorders. Similarly, the loss of tolerance to certain self antigens appears to be important in many disorders. This process could occur as a result of cross sensitivity to foreign antigens or alteration of native antigens. T-lymphocytic cells termed "helper cells" appear to be instrumental in promoting B-cell reactivity responsible for antibody production. Similarly, T-"suppressor" cells may be deficient in regulating the excess production of antibodies by B-cells.

REF: Rabin, B.S. and Winkelstein, A. "Theories of auto-immunity." Bull Rheum Dis 26:3, 842-847, 1975-76.

273. Q. In the context of newer data available on the interaction of T- and B-lymphocytes in autoimmune disorders, comment on the present techniques of therapy and what appear to be the trends for future therapy in these disorders.

A. Treatment of the autoimmune disorders such as systemic lupus erythematosus, rheumatoid arthritis, and so on has concentrated either on suppressing the inflammatory response once it has been initiated, or suppressing the immunological system that gave rise to the inflammatory reaction in the first place. Thus, antiinflammatory drugs and immunosuppressive medications have formed the basis of therapy in these disorders. However, it is entirely possible that more promising patterns of treatment will emerge based on immunostimulation (of suppressor lymphocytes) rather than immunosuppression. Preliminary work with immunostimulants in rheumatoid arthritis has yielded encouraging clinical data. Similarly, it has been predicted that techniques will emerge that would eliminate cross reacting or altered self antigens, or would restore tolerance to critical self antigens where this tolerance has been lost.

REF: Rabin, B.S. and Winkelstein, A. "Theories of auto-immunity." Bull Rheum Dis 26:3, 842-847, 1975-76.

274. Q. What are the four types of specific allergic reactions responsible for hypersensitivity disorders of the lungs?

A. The four types of allergic pulmonary hypersensitivity disorders that have been described are (1) the IgE dependent reagin mediated reaction, (2) the cytotoxic, tissue specific antibody mediated type, (3) immune complex disease, and (4) cell mediated or delayed hypersensitivity reactions.

REF: McCombs, R. P. "Diseases due to immunologic reactions in the lungs (First of two parts)." New Engl J Med 286:22 1185-11250, 1972.

275. Q. Describe IgE and list the various types of disorders wherein you would expect this antibody to be significantly elevated.

A. IgE is an immunoglobulin that has also been called reagin or reaginic antibody. It is a glycoprotein with a sedimentation coefficient of 8.2 and appears to be responsible for skin sensitization. The typical serum concentration is between 100 and 700 ng per milliliter. The half life is only two days or so. Increased levels of IgE are seen in asthma, eczema, allergic rhinitis, certain types of food sensitivities, parasitic infections, allergic aspergillosis, and other disorders.

REF: McCombs, R. P. "Diseases due to immunologic reactions in the lungs (First of two parts)." New Engl J Med 286:22, 1185-1250, 1972.

276. Q. What is meant by the term "immunologic surveillance" as described by Burnet in 1970 ?

A. The central issue of this concept is that it is up to the immune system to recognize and ultimately destroy cancer cells while they are still in the early stages of formation. If this process is competent, then it is argued that neoplasia will not appear. However, when this process breaks down, then the stage is set for the development of malignant disease.

REF: Schwartz, R.S. "Another look at immunologic surveillance." New Engl J Med 293:4, 181-184, 1975.

Burnet, F.M. "The concept of immunological surveillance." Prog Exp Tumor Res 13:1-27, 1970.

277. Q. What is the status of Burnet's theory of "immunological surveillance" in the light of current concepts?

A. Although many experimental lines of research lend
support to this concept of pathogenesis, there are also additional lines of data that suggest other aspects of the immune system as being of prime importance. For instance,
it is well known that some disorders that involve anergy,
such as leprosy and sarcoidosis do not seem to be associated
with an increased incidence of neoplasia. Certain tumors
appear to require antibody enhancement in order to prolif-
erate. It is these and other concepts that have perhaps
shifted the emphasis away from immune surveillance to
such areas as immunostimulation. In this context, it has
been proposed that the future of research in this area is in
terms of neither immune suppression or stimulation, but
rather immunoregulation.

REF: Schwartz, R. S. "Another look at immunologic surveillance." New Engl J Med 293:4, 181-184, 1975.

278. Q. Immune complex glomerulonephritis may occur in
a wide variety of viral, bacterial, and parasitic disorders.
Name some of these disorders and comment as to which disorder has been associated with the finding of the causative
organism in the glomerular lesion.

A. In the nephrotic syndrome due to malaria, the
presence of the malarial organism in the glomerulus has
been definitely established. In other instances of glomerulonephritis due to infecting organisms, the presence of the
antigenic material as originating from the infecting organism has been more inferential. These disorders include
streptococcal glomerulonephritis, hepatitis-B associated
glomerulonephritis, leprosy, secondary syphilis, bacterial
endocarditis, infections of arteriovenous shunts, and more
recently, with schistosomiasis.

REF: Falcao, H. A., and Gould, D. B. "Immune complex
nephropathy in schistosomiasis." Ann Intern Med 83,
148-154, 1975.

279. Q. In studies of delayed hypersensitivity in rheumatic
diseases, what general conclusions can be drawn on the
basis of currently available data?

A. Studies with lymphocytic reactivity in systemic
lupus erythematosus, rheumatoid arthritis, progressive
systemic sclerosis, and other connective tissue disorders,
it appears that patients with systemic lupus erythematosus
and rheumatoid arthritis appear to have impaired lymphocyte responsiveness as measured by mitogen stimulation.
Treatment did not affect this responsiveness. The conclusion that has been drawn in the context of this and similar
other data is that there is good probability that patients with
SLE and rheumatoid arthritis have a specific cellular immunodeficiency state which may facilitate the development
of clinical mnaifestations.

REF: Lockshin, M.D., Eisenhauer, A.C., Kohn, R.,
et. al. "Cell mediated immunity in rheumatic diseases."
Arth Rheum 18:3, 245-250, 1975.

280. Q. In the study of lymphocytic function as defined by
mitogen responsiveness, production of MIF, and delayed
hypersensitivity, what patterns of response would you expect to see with active systemic lupus erythematosus, minimally active disease, and patients with discoid lupus? What
is the effect of DNA as an antigen in blast transformation
in these groups?

A. The more active patients with systemic lupus erythematosus appeared to have a greater impairment of lymphocyte function as measured by these various parameters.
In contrast, patients with mild forms of the disease, or
with discoid lupus did not appear to differ greatly from control groups. DNA did not appear to act as an immunostimulant to lymphocytes in these patients and had no effect on
blast transformation.

REF: Rosenthal, C.J. and Franklin, E.C. "Depression of
cellular mediated immunity in systemic lupus erythematosus."
Arth Rheum 18:3, 207-217, 1975.

281. Q. Comment on antilymphocyte antibodies in systemic lupus erythematosus, their significance, and what effect might be seen in T and B cell enumeration studies?

A. Although antibodies against lymphocytes in systemic lupus erythematosus may cause lymphopenia, they need not necessarily be associated with lymphocytotoxic activity. Although the enumeration of T-cells will not be affected by such antibodies, the determination of B-cells by the technique of surface immunoglobulin assay will be influenced by antilymphocyte antibodies in SLE.

REF: Messner, R. P., Kennedy, M. S., and Jelinek, J. G. "Antilymphocyte antibodies in systemic lupus erythematosus." Arth Rheum 18:3, 201-206, 1975.

282. Q. In the rheumatoid synovial membrane, what type of lymphocyte is most frequently found and what are the potential mechanisms of action that have been suggested for this lymphocyte?

A. Approximately 80 to 85% of the lymphocytes found in the synovial tissue of rheumatoid arthritis are T-cells as judged by the sheep cell rosette formation technique. Although the precise role of these T-cells is unknown, it has been speculated that they may be cytotoxic effector cells, "helper cells" augmenting antibody mediated tissue injury, or releasers of lymphokines that in turn promote tissue damage and eventual fibrosis.

REF: Bankhurst, A. D., Husby, G., and Williams, R. C., Jr. "Predominance of T cells in the lymphocytic infiltrates of synovial tissues in rheumatoid arthritis." Arth Rheum 19:3, 555-562, 1976.

283. Q. Define "autoimmune disease."

A. An autoimmune disease is one wherein the pathological process depends primarily on an immunological mechanism that has been initiated by humoral or cellular events directed against self antigens which previously enjoyed tolerance.

REF: Rabin, B. S. and Winkelstein, A. "Theories of Autoimmunity." Bull Rheum Dis 26:3, 842-847, 1975-76.

284. Q. Discuss Witebsky's postulates and comment as to the feasibility of demonstrating these postulates in the various connective tissue disorders such as systemic lupus erythematosus, rheumatoid arthritis, and so forth.

A. The criteria for autoimmunity described by Witebsky and Milgrom are the following: (1) the presence of antibody or cellular specificity against tissue of the target organ, (2) the identification of an antigen within the target organ against which the antibody and cellular system is directed, (3) when animals are immunized with this antigen, an appropriate immune response should be elicited, which (4) will then produce the disease in question, (5) transfer of the disease state with antibodies or immunocompetent cells is possible from one experimental animal to another. Although several clinical disorders thought of as being autoimmune in nature meet one or more of these postulates, there is no disorder that meets all five. Furthermore, it is speculated that it may be impossible to meet all five postulates in view of the enormous complexity and the multifactorial nature of the connective tissue and autoimmune disorders.

REF: Rabin, B.S. and Winkelstein, A. "Theories of autoimmunity." Bull Rheum Dis 26:3, 842-847, 1975-76.

285. Q. What effects have been noted in NZB mice treated with levamisole and comment on the implications for future directions regarding research and treatment in human systemic lupus erythematosus?

A. Whereas immunosuppressive medications such as azathioprine and cyclophosphamide have been used almost exclusively to suppress the clinical and laboratory features of lupus in the NZB mouse model, recent attention has turned to immunostimulants such as levamisole on the assumption that deficient cellular function is perhaps responsible for enhanced humoral responsiveness. Hence, by stimulating the deficient population of T-cells that presumably is no longer restraining the B-cell lines from producing antibody, clinical and laboratory improvement will result. In studies with NZB mice a significant effect was observed with levamisole in delaying mortality, the development of antinuclear antibodies, and proteinuria.

REF: Russell, A. S. "Therapeutic trials with levamisole and other agents in NZB mice." J Rheum 3:4, 380-383, 1976.

286. Q. Discuss the sensitivity and specificity of various antinuclear antibodies in systemic lupus erythematosus.

A. Antinuclear antibodies may occur in various forms in systemic lupus erythematosus. Antibody to deoxyribonucleoprotein (DNP) reaches a 98% sensitivity in SLE with however, a relatively high overlap with other connective tissue disorders and chronic active hepatitis, wherein it is found in 15 to 40% of cases. The single stranded (denatured) anti-DNA is positive in greater than 90% of patients with SLE, but also positive in 20 to 60% of patients with other connective tissue disorders and chronic active hepatitis, much as is the case for the DNP test. Antibodies to native (double stranded) DNA are highly specific for SLE, particularly lupus nephritis, and especially when present in relatively high titers. Only 3 to 9% of patients with rheumatoid arthritis will demonstrate anti-native DNA titers. However, the native DNA titer is unfortunately not very sensitive in that only 40 to 60% of patients with active lupus will demonstrate high titers. Similarly, the Sm-(RNAase resistant ENA) antigen is present almost exclusively in lupus, but is of relatively low sensitivity (30%).

REF: McDuffie, F. C. and Bunch, T. W. "Immunologic tests in the diagnosis of rheumatic diseases." Bull Rheum Dis 27:5, 900-905, 1976-77.

287. Q. Discuss the sensitivity and specificity of antinuclear antibodies with a nucleolar pattern in the diagnosis of progressive systemic sclerosis.

A. When the antibody to nucleoli is found in significant titer producing a positive antinuclear antibody test with a nucleolar pattern, this becomes a relatively specific finding serologically for progressive systemic sclerosis. Only 5% or less of other connective tissue disorders, including systemic lupus erythematosus, demonstrate elevated titers of this specificity. However, the degree of sensitivity is very low, limiting the usefulness of this as a diagnostic test in progressive systemic sclerosis. Only 20% of patients with PSS have positive antinuclear antibody titers of a nucleolar pattern.

REF: McDuffie, F.C. and Bunch, T.W. "Immunologic tests in the diagnosis of rheumatic diseases." Bull Rheum Dis 27:5, 900-905, 1976-77.

288. Q. What techniques are currently available to measure and detect the presence of immune complexes in serum? Comment on their relative usefulness.

A. Initial techniques of determining the presence of immune complexes depended on difficult and semiquantitative measures such as the release of histamine in guinea pig lung when perfused with serum containing immune complex material, or inferences drawn from decreased serum complement levels assumed to be fixed by immune complex formation. However, more recent advances have now enabled rather direct quantification of immune complexes by such techniques as (1) the Clq precipitin test, (2) monoclonal rheumatoid factor radioimmunoassay, and the (3) C receptor lymphocyte test (Raji cell test). In general, there is relatively good agreement between these tests when measuring immune complex material. However, for certain reasons that have yet to be fully elucidated, one test will detect a certain type of immune complex while another test will fail to do so.

REF: McDuffie, F.C. and Bunch, T.W. "Immunologic tests in the diagnosis of rheumatic diseases." Bull Rheum Dis 27:6, 906-911, 1976-77.

289. Q. Name the congenital disorders associated with cell mediated immunodeficiency states.

A. The various congenital disorders wherein cellular immunity is either lacking or deficient include: DiGeorge syndrome (thymic hypoplasia), Nezelhof syndrome (autosomal recessive lymphopenia), cartilage hair hypoplasia, chronic mucocutaneous candidiasis, Wiskott-Aldrich syndrome (immunodeficiency with thrombocytopenia), ataxia telangiectasia, and severe combined deficiency disease.

REF: Wing, E.J. and Remington, J.S. "Cell mediated immunity and its role in resistance to infection." West J Med 126, 14-31, 1977.

290. Q. Name the viral, bacterial, and fungal infections that appear to be associated with defects in delayed type hypersensitivity.

A. Various viral illnesses such as measles, mumps, chicken pox, influenza, infectious mononucleosis, yellow fever, and rubella, as well as measles, mumps, rubella vaccine, have been associated with deficient delayed type hypersensitivity. The bacterial infections include tuberculosis, leprosy, syphilis, streptococcal infections, brucellosis, typhoid fever, and various pneumonias. The fungal disorders include coccidioidomycosis, histoplasmosis, and blastomycosis.

REF: Wing, E.J. and Remington, J.S. "Cell mediated immunity and its role in resistance to infection." West J Med 126, 14-31, 1977.

291. Q. Discuss the various systemic disorders and other significant factors with the exception of medications and drugs that depress cell mediated immunity.

A. Aside from drugs such as corticosteroids and immunosuppressives, certain systemic illnesses may result in disorders of delayed type hypersensitivity. These include malnutrition, diabetes mellitus, uremia, surgery and anesthesia, sarcoidosis, and heroin addiction. Age is also a significant factor in the development of depressed cell mediated immunity. In contrast, the frequency of autoantibodies such as the rheumatoid factor, antinuclear antibody, and so forth appears to increase with age.

REF: Wing, E.J. and Remington, J.S. "Cell mediated immunity and its role in resistance to infection." West J Med 126, 14-31, 1977.

292. Q. Discuss the presence of immune complexes in infective endocarditis before and after appropriate antibiotic or surgical treatment.

A. Up to 97% of patients with infective endocarditis demonstrated significantly elevated levels of immune complexes in their serum as measured by the Raji cell radioimmune assay. Immune complexes were correlated with decreased serum complement, longer duration of disease, right sided endocarditis, extravascular manifestations, and positive blood cultures. With treatment, the level of immune complexes dropped to zero with a rise in serum complement, improvement in the extravascular manifestations, and the appearance of negative blood cultures.

REF: Vayer, A.S., Theofilopoulos, A.N., Eisenberg, R., et.al. "Circulating immune complexes in infective endocarditis." New Engl J Med 295:27, 1500-1504, 1976.

293. Q. In bone marrow transplantation among HLA identical siblings, what are the most significant factors that will influence eventual successful engraftment and survival?

A. In a study of 73 consecutive HLA identical sibling bone marrow transplantations, it was concluded that the two most significant variables affecting engraftment and survival were (1) a positive mixed leukocyte culture and (2) a low number of donor marrow cells. When these elements were noted, poor survival resulted. Therefore, it would appear important to emphasize the need for complete and thorough immunosuppression together with transplantation of the greatest amount of donor marrow available.

REF: Storb, R., Prentice, R.L., and Thomas, E.D., "Marrow transplantation for treatment of aplastic anemia." New Engl J Med 296:2, 61-66, 1977.

294. Q. Discuss IgD as a surface immunoglobulin and its possible significance.

A. IgD is a carbohydrate rich antibody molecule with two H and two L chains. It has been found on lymphocyte membranes as a surface antigen both in normal as well as abnormal lymphocytic cells. Although its function is still speculative, it has been proposed that IgD may have an important role in antigen recognition and subsequent modulation of the immune response.

REF: Franklin, E. C. "Some impacts of clinical investigation on immunology." New Engl J Med 294:10, 531-537, 1976.

295. Q. Monoclonal antibody specificity has been associated with what disorders?

A. Lymphocytes from patients with chronic lymphocytic leukemia, Waldenstrom's macroglobulinemia, and certain other forms of lymphoma appear to bear monoclonal immunoglobulins usually of both the IgD as well as the IgG type. Occasionally, the monoclonal antibody will be of one or the other type of immunoglobulin. This is in contrast to acute lymphocytic leukemia and multiple myeloma which do not bear surface immunoglobulins. Hence, it can be said that lymphocytes derived from Waldenstrom's macroglobulinemia and CLL are B-cell type.

REF: Franklin, E. C. "Some impacts of clinical investigation on immunology." New Engl J Med 294:10, 531-537, 1976.

296. Q. Describe the sequence of events involved in the induction of atopic hypersensitivity by the IgE molecule.

A. Mast cells and basophils have Fc fragment receptors on their membrane surfaces which react with the Fc-fragment of the IgE antibody molecule. When such a reaction takes place, degranulation of the mast cell and basophil occurs with release of vasoactive substances such as histamine, serotonin, and slow reacting substance-A.

REF: Franklin, E. C. "Some impacts of clinical investigation on immunology." New Engl J Med 294:10, 531-537, 1976.

297. Q. The role of IgE has been clearly defined in the causation of atopic disorders and allergic asthma. However, a more positive role for this antibody has yet to be elucidated, although one would assume some beneficial effect

would have to be present to perpetuate its presence on an evolutionary level. Consider some of the possible roles of IgE in this latter context that have been proposed.

A. IgE bound to mast cells and basophils may increase vascular permeability enabling other antibodies to more easily reach tissue sites otherwise inaccessible to them. The cytophilic properties of IgE for macrophages has led to the speculation that IgE may be involved in the killing function of these cells. But perhaps the most intriguing data is found in various parasitic infections such as schistosomiasis where evidence is emerging that suggests an enhancement of IgG mediated killing of these infective organisms.

REF: Franklin, E. C. "Some impacts of clinical investigation on immunology." New Engl J Med 294:10, 531-537, 1976.

298. Q. What disorders are associated with monoclonal immunoglobulins?

A. Multiple myeloma, Waldenstrom's macroblobulinemia, amyloidosis, heavy chain disease, and genetically induced or sporadic instances of monoclonal gammopathy may be seen. In addition, autoimmune disorders, carcinomatosis, liver disease, and chronic inflammatory disease of various organ systems may produce monoclonal immunoglobulins.

REF: Zawadski, Z. A., and Edwards, G. A. "Clinical significance of monoclonal immunoglobulinemia." Bull Rheum Dis 25:6, 810-815, 1974-75.

299. Q. What are the laboratory findings that would suggest the presence of a malignant gammopathy?

A. If the serum M component is at a concentration that is greater than 2 g per dl for IgG, or 1 g per dl for IgM or IgA, or if Bence-Jones proteinuria is demonstrable by the heat test, these findings suggest a malignant condition. Further "warning signs" include: progressive increase in the concentration of the M-component, decreased

levels of normal immunoglobulins, hyperviscosity, hypoal-
buminemia, marrow plasmacytosis with atypical or im-
mature forms, and decreased B-lymphocytes in the peripheral
blood.

REF: Zawadzki, Z.A. and Edwards, G.A. "Clinical significance of monoclonal immunoglobulinemia." Bull Rheum
Dis 25:6, 810-815, 1974-75.

300. Q. If you, as a physician, are presented with a patient
who is found to have a monoclonal immunoglobulin on serum
electrophoresis, what diagnostic steps should be taken to
properly evaluate such a patient?

A. The paraprotein should be confirmed and characterized by monovalent antisera for light and heavy chains.
Serum viscosity, cryoglobulin determination, and charac-
terization of the paraprotein as possibly being a cold aglu-
tinin should be performed. Comprehensive diagnostic
studies for myeloma or carinomatosis should be conducted,
and long term follow up instituted with serial examinations
of the serum or urine electrophoretically, bone marrow
examination, hematologic parameters, and skeletal radiographs. Treatment for assymptomatic monoclonal
immunoglobulinemia should be avoided.

REF: Zawadzki, Z.A. and Edwards, G.A. "Clinical significance of monoclonal immunoglobulinemia." Bull Rheum
Dis 25:6, 810-815, 1974-75.

301. Q. Discuss secretory immunoglobulins and their
proposed biologic role.

A. Although IgA represents a small fraction of serum
immunoglobulins, it is the predominant species in external
secretions such as the saliva, gastrointestinal fluid, and
so forth. IgA is probably produced locally in the lamina
propria of the mucous membrane or gladular tissue. The
proposed biologic role for IgA is that of protecting against
viral infections at mucous membranes of the respiratory
tract, gastrointestinal tract, and so forth.

REF: Tomasi, T.B., Jr. "Secretory immunoglobulins."
New Engl J Med 287:10, 500-506, 1972.

302. Q. Discuss the types of chronic polyarthritis that have been described in hypogammaglobulinemia and immunodeficiency states.

A. A syndrome similar to rheumatoid arthritis has been described in patients with hypogammaglobulinemia. Histologically, the synovium in such patients reveals changes typical of those that might be seen in rheumatoid arthritis or in any inflammatory chronic synovitis. Small levels of immunoglobulin may be found in the synovium or in the synovial fluid. However, in other patients the chronic synovitis appears to arise in the absence of B-cells or detectable levels of immunoglobulins in the synovium. The histological pattern in these cases does not resemble that seen in rheumatoid arthritis.

REF: Grayzel, A. I. , Marcus, R. , Stern, R. , and Winchester, R. J. "Chronic polyarthritis associated with hypogammaglobulinemia." Arth Rheum 20:3, 887-894, 1977.

303. Q. Discuss cryglobulins in vasculitis.

A. Cryoglobulinemia may be detected in approximately 30% of patients with certain types of chronic vasculitic skin lesions. Cryoblobulins have also been detected in certain types of glomerulonephritis, systemic lupus erythematosus, and other types of immunological disorders. Generally, the cryoglobulins are either IgA or IgM which are directed against IgG and which exist in immune complexes. Serum complement levels in uncomplicated vasculitis remain normal, although in glomerulonephritis, the serum complement may decrease.

REF: Cream, J. J. "Cryoglobulins in vasculitis." Clin ex Immunol 10, 117-126, 1972.

304. Q. Name the activators of the properdin or alternative pathway in the complement system.

A. Properdin has been shown to be activated by complex polysacchardies such as zymosan, bacterial cell wall products and endotoxin, during gram negative bacteremia wherein the biologically active products so released may contribute to the development of shock, and IgA containing complexes.

REF: Fearon, D. T. , Ruddy, S. , Schur, P. H. , and McCabe, W. R. "Activation of the properdin pathway of complement in patients with gram negative bacteremia." New Engl J Med 292:18, 937-940, 1975.

XIII. ANTIINFLAMMATORY AND IMMUNOSUPPRESSIVE
DRUGS IN THE TREATMENT OF RHEUMATIC
DISORDERS

305. Q. In the treatment of rheumatoid arthritis, what is
the relationship of serum gold levels to the therapeutic
response?

A. Most of the studies in the literature regarding serum gold levels and therapeutic effectiveness suggest that
there is no consistent relationship between the serum gold
level and the therapeutic response. The minimal dose of
gold sodium thiomalate required to produce a therapeutic
response is on the order of 25 mgm or less per week. However, in a study that measured therapeutic response in patients whose steady-state gold level varied from 95 to 386
micrograms/dl no significant differences were noted between
patients with higher gold levels as opposed to those with
lower levels.

REF: Sharp, J.T., Lidsky, M.D., Duffy, J., et.al. "Comparison of two dosage schedules of gold salts in the treatment of rheumatoid arthritis." Arth Rheum 20:6, 1179-
1187, 1977.

306. Q. What is the effect of aspirin on delayed hypersensitivity?

A. Treatment with aspirin in doses upto 4 gm daily
appears to produce no significant effect on delayed hypersensitivity as measured by skin test reactivity, lymphocyte
proliferation, and the percentage of T-lymphocytes.

REF: Duncan, M.W., Person, D.A., Rich, R.R. and Sharp,
J.T. "Aspirin and delayed type hypersensitivity." Arth
Rheum 20:6, 1174-1178, 1977.

307. Q. Discuss the relationship of the mechanism of action
of the various nonsteroidal antiinflammatory agents to
prostaglandin biosynthesis.

A. It is currently hypothesized that aspirin and the
nonsteroidal antiinflammatory drugs such as indomethacin

exert their pharmacological actions by inhibiting prostaglandin synthesis. The data suggest that these drugs act by becoming competitive-irreversible inhibitors and that in all likelihood these drugs block an early, and possibly the initial, stage of prostaglandin synthesis.

REF: Tomlinson, R. V., Ringold, H. J., Qureshi, M. C., and Forchielli, E. "Relationship between inhibition of prostaglandin synthesis and drug efficacy: support for the current theory of the mode of action of aspirin-like drugs." Biochemical and biophysical research communications, 46:552-559, 1972.

308. Q. Discuss the mechanisms postulated for penicillamine in the treatment of rheumatoid arthritis.

A. The previously held theory that penicillamine exerts its therapeutic effect in rheumatoid arthritis by splitting the IgM rheumatoid factor is no longer acceptable. Conflicting experimental data regarding penicillamine as an immunosuppressive drug exist. Several studies suggest that penicillamine exerts an immunosuppressive effect, and still other studies suggest an enhanced immune response. Therefore, the role of penicillamine in the immune response is unclear. Another mechanism of action that has been suggested for penicillamine is that it may inhibit binding of complement to immunoglobulins in immune complexes.

REF: Mellbye, O. J. and Munthe, E. "Effect of penicillamine on complement in vitro and in vivo." Ann Rheum Dis 36:453-458, 1977.

309. Q. What is the expected response rate and the frequency of complications in rheumatoid arthritis patients treated with penicillamine?

A. Objective clinical improvement was noted in approximately 65% of patients by the conventional parameters while adverse reactions occurred in 49% of patients. The most common complications included skin rashes, taste disturbances, gastrointestinal irritation, and proteinuria. In a group of 179 patients studied in a multi-center trial, no serious side effects such as bone marrow toxicity were reported.

REF: Shiokawa, Y., Horiuchi, Y. Honma, M., et.al. "Clinical evaluation of D-Penicillamine by multicentric double-blind comparative study in chronic rheumatoid arthritis." Arth and Rheum, 20:8, 1464-1472, 1977.

310. Q. What is the role of levamisole in rheumatoid arthritis and is there a beneficial therapeutic effect as judged by controlled clinical trials?

A. Levamisole is an antheliminthic drug which has the properties of stimulating cell mediated immunity and macrophage function. This is in contrast to many other types of treatments for rheumatoid arthritis which have a suppressive effect on immunological function, such as corticosteroid medication and cytotoxic agents. In a double-blind controlled study, significant improvement was noted as compared to a placebo control group. Adverse side effects were relatively few and limited essentially to mild alterations in taste.

REF: Runge, L.A., Pinals, R.S., Lourie, S.H., and Tomar, R.H., "Treatment of rheumatoid arthritis with levamisole." Arth and Rheum 20:8, 1445-1448, 1977.

311. Q. What is the projected role of penicillamine in the treatment of rheumatoid arthritic patients who either fail to improve with a gold program or who exhibit unacceptable side effects from gold?

A. In a study of 44 patients who developed significant side effects from gold or who failed to respond to a gold program, the use of penicillamine demonstrated encouraging therapeutic improvement in most patients considered chrysotherapy "failures." The pattern of toxicity with penicillamine was independent of that seen with gold suggesting that the drug could be used safely in patients reacting adversely to gold. However, toxicity from penicillamine proved significant requiring discontinuation of the drug in 25% of patients due to mucocutaneous, renal, or hematologic complications. This was despite the "go-low, go-slow" method of administration.

REF: Tsang, I.K., Patterson, C.A., Stein, H.B., et.al. "D-Penicillamine in the treatment of rheumatoid arthritis." Arth Rheum 20:2, 666-670, 1977.

312. Q. In a patient on corticosteroid medication in whom rapid reduction in the dosage is undertaken, what are the typical symptoms and signs that can be anticipated?

A. The typical signs of corticosteroid withdrawal are as follows: weakness, fatigue, arthralgia, nausea, anorexia, dizziness, orthostatic hypotension, dyspnea, hypoglycemia, and desquamation of the skin.

REF: Byyny, R.L. "Withdrawal from glucocorticoid therapy." New Engl J Med 295:11, 30-32, 1976.

313. Q. Discuss the pharmacology of indomethacin serum levels in patients treated with this drug.

A. The serum level of indomethacin rises rapidly in fasting subjects taking the drug orally. Within 30 to 90 minutes, peak serum levels are identified. Food and antacids reduce the peak concentration of the drug. Steady state serum levels occur after 24 hours. When indomethacin is given as 25 mgm every four hours as compared to 50 mgm every eight hours, the peak concentrations are similar, but the average concentrations of the drug are greater and the fluctuations in the serum level are smaller when the more frequent dosage schedule is selected.

REF: Emori, H.W., Paulus, H., Bluestone, R., et.al. "Indomethacin serum concentrations in man." Ann Rheum Dis 35, 333-338, 1976.

314. Q. Explain the relevance of enzyme induction in a patient on corticosteroid medication.

A. Certain drugs may alter the hepatic metabolism of a number of drugs such as corticosteroids. The list of agents capable of causing the process of hepatic enzyme induction is lengthy and includes barbiturates, diphenylhydantoin, glutethimide, meprobamate, phenylbutazone, tolbutamide, and ethanol. In a patient on corticosteroid medication, the addition of a drug capable of causing enzyme induction in the liver, could theoretically lead to enhanced clearance of corticosteroid preparation thereby resulting in deterioration of the patient's clinical status. This factor can be significant in a patient on multiple drug regimens.

REF: Brooks, P.M., Buchanan, W.W., Grove, M., and Downie, W.W. "Effects of enzyme induction on metabolism of prednisolone." Ann Rheum Dis 35, 339-343, 1976.

315. Q. At what point would one expect some degree of suppression of the hypothalamic-pituitary-adrenal axis in a patient being given corticosteroid medication? What are the factors that govern adrenal suppression?

A. The degree of suppression of the hypothalamic-pituitary-adrenal axis depends on the dose of medication given, the frequency and route of administration, the duration of treatment, and the type of corticosteroid drug selected. Corticosteroid medication given in a dosage range that does not exceed the equivalent of prednisone, 40 mgm daily in a single morning-administration will not produce appreciable adrenal suppression for the first 5-7 days. However, longer courses with smaller doses, or shorter courses with higher doses will generally result in suppression of adrenal function. Alternate-day treatment with doses of prednisone under 40 mgm generally produces little in the way of significant adrenal suppression.

REF: Byyny, R.L. "Withdrawal from glucocorticosteroid therapy." New Engl J Med 295:1, 30-32, 1976.

316. Q. Describe the procedure that a physician might follow in withdrawing corticosteroid medication in a patient who has been treated with corticosteroid drugs for a long period of time.

A. When corticosteroid medication is tapered, the physician must watch for evidence of increased activity of the systemic disease as well as for symptoms of withdrawal.

In general, the hypothalamic and pituitary limbs of the system recovery prior to the adrenal cortex, which tends to recover last. The initial step in the tapering process is to bring the dosage of corticosteroid medication to a "physiological" dosage which would mean 20 mgm of hydrocortisone, 5 mgm of prednisone or prednisolone, and 0.75 mgm of dexamethasone. When this is accomplished, the patient can be switched from whatever type of steroid that has been given to hydrocortisone 20 mgm as a single morning-administration. Tapering is then conducted at a rate of 2.5 mgm weekly to a total dose of 10 mgm hydrocortisone. Monthly serum cortisol determinations are obtained at 8 a.m. which should exceed 10 micrograms per 100 ml before the physician can conclude that baseline pituitary-adrenal function is adequate. A short ACTH test will verify that adrenal reserve is adequate if after a single intramuscular injection of cosyntropin, 250 micrograms, the plasma cortisol rises in 30 to 60 minutes to either 20 micrograms per 100 ml or the increment from baseline in 6 micrograms per 100 ml.

REF: Byyny, D. L. "Withdrawal from glucocorticoid therapy." New Engl J Med 295:1, 30-32, 1976.

317. Q. What significance would you attribute to the development of eosinophilia in a patient on chrysotherapy?

A. Adverse clinical reactions to gold injections have been associated with the development of eosinophilia and increased serum IgE levels. These parameters return to normal after the gold has been discontinued and the adverse reaction has disappeared. Because IgE has been implicated, it is possible that adverse reactions to gold may be mediated by a type-I hypersensitivity mechanism. Skin reactions appear to be the most common type of adverse effect associated with eosinophilia.

REF: Davis, P., and Hughes, G.R.V. "Significance of eosionophilia during gold therapy." Arth and Rheum 17:6, 964-968, 1974.

318. Q. Categorize the more commonly used corticosteroid agents into "short-acting," "intermediate," and "long-acting" preparations and state the approximate equivalent dosages.

A. The "short-acting" corticosteroid drugs are cortisol (hydrocortisone) (20 mgm); cortisone (25 mgm); prednisone

(5 mgm); prednisolone (5 mgm); methylprednisolone (4 mgm). The "intermediate" corticosteroid in most common use is triamcinolone (4 mgm). The "long-acting" drugs are betamethasone (0.60 mgm) and dexamethasone (0.75 mgm).

REF: Axelrod, L. "Glucocorticoid therapy." Medicine 55:1, 39-65, 1976.

319. Q. What important considerations should you as a physician review when considering the use of glucocorticoids?

A. Glucocorticoid drugs are "two-edged swords" capable of numerous side effects as well as possessing considerable therapeutic efficacy. Important considerations in their use would include the seriousness of the disorder to be treated; the length of time therapy will be required; the anticipated dosage that will be necessary to control the disease process; the presence of certain relative "contraindications" to steroidal therapy (diabetes mellitus, osteoporosis, peptic ulcer disease, gastritis, esophagitis, tuberculosis or other chronic infections, hypertension and cardiovascular disease, psychological difficulties); alternative modes of treatment; which type of corticosteroid should be selected; and whether an alternate-day schedule of administration would be indicated.

REF: Axelrod, L. "Glucocorticoid therapy." Medicine 55:1, 39-65, 1976.

320. Q. Compare and contrast naturally occurring Cushing's syndrome with iatrogenic Cushing's syndrome as to signs and symptoms.

A. Both naturally occurring and iatrogenic Cushing's syndrome feature obesity, psychiatric symptoms, edema, and poor wound-healing. However, in iatrogenic Cushing's syndrome the following are virtually unique: benign intracranial hypertension, glaucoma, posterior subscapular cataracts, pancreatitis, aseptic necrosis of bone, and panniculitis. In naturally occurring Cushing's syndrome, the following are characteristic: hypertension, acne, menstrual disturbances or impotence in males, hirsutism or virilism, striae, purpura, and plethora.

REF: Axelrod, L. "Glucocorticoid therapy." Medicine 55:1, 39-65, 1976.

321. Q. Describe the effects of corticosteroid drugs on inflammation and immunologically-mediated disease processes.

A. Glucocorticosteroids result in the production of a neutrophilic leukocytosis together with a lymphocytopenia, eosinopenia, and monocytopenia. The T-lymphocytic population is especially prone to the effects of corticosteroid drugs. It is believed that the lymphocytopenia results from a redistribution of lymphocytes, rather than direct lysis of these cells. Certain modifications of lymphocyte function have also been attributed to corticosteroid medication. These include diminished delayed-hypersensitivity response; decreased access of lymphocytic cells to antigen; decreased antigen-induced blastogenesis; reduced macrophage responsiveness to MIF and MAF; and evidence of target-cell protection in cell-mediated cytotoxicity studies. Additionally, corticosteroids delay the migration of neutrophils and monocytes to areas of inflammation, and this appears to be one of the more important effects of glucocorticoids in suppressing inflammation.

REF: Fauci, A.S., Dale, D.C., and Balow, J.E. "Glucocorticosteroid therapy: mechanisms of action and clinical considerations." Ann Intern Med 84:304-315, 1976.

322. Q. Discuss the hepatotoxicity of aspirin.

A. Salicylates are mildly hepatotoxic in some people Usually the transaminases are affected. Patients with systemic lupus erythematosus appear to be somewhat more vulnerable to the hepatotoxic effects of aspirin, although other disorders such as rheumatoid arthritis, juvenile rheumatoid arthritis, and normal individuals also may develop liver function abnormalities. Permanent liver disease does not appear to develop.

REF: Seaman, W.E. and Plotz, P.H. "Effect of aspirin on liver tests in patients with RA or SLE and in normal volunteers." Arth Rheum 19:2, 155-160, 1976.

323. Q. Describe the histological changes known to occur in the gastric mucosa with aspirin ingestion.

A. When aspirin is ingested orally, there is evidence of disruption of the mucosal barrier in the stomach. Ten minutes after ingestion, 25% of surface epithelial cells on gastric biopsy reveal evidence of mucosal damage. The changes noted include focal cell disruption, loss of granules from the gastric mucosa, membrane rupture, and honey-combing. In 1 hour, these changes regress markedly.

REF: Baskin, W.N., Ivey, K.J., Krause, W.J., et.al. "Aspirin-induced ultrastructural changes in human gastric mucosa." Ann Intern Med 85:299-303, 1976.

324. Q. In a patient who develops heavy proteinuria while on penicillamine for treatment of rheumatoid arthritis, what would be the immunopathology of a renal biopsy?

A. The histological picture in penicillamine-induced proteinuria is generally focal proliferative or membranous glomerulonephritis with subepithelial electron-dense deposits. The renal biopsy may also appear normal. Immunofluorescent staining reveals immune-complex deposits of IgG, IgM, and C3. Although antibodies have been found to penicillamine in the serum, elution techniques have failed to identify penicillamine in the renal glomerulus and the nature of the antigen therefore remains unknown.

REF: Dische, F.E., Swinson, D.R., Hamilton, E.B.D., and Parsons, V. "Immunopathology of penicillamine-induced glomerular disease." J of Rheum 3:2, 145-154, 1976.

325. Q. Discuss the interaction of nonsteroidal antiinflammatory agents with aspirin and the clinical significance in patients treated with combination therapy.

A. When nonsteroidal antiinflammatory agents such as naproxen, fenoprofen, and indomethacin are given with aspirin, the serum drug levels of the non-steroidal agent are generally reduced when compared to serum levels of these drugs when given alone. The serum salicylate level remains unaffected. However, the clinical significance of these observations remains unclear. Although the serum drug levels have been found to be lower with combination therapy, some studies have suggested a synergistic effect with aspirin.

REF: Rubin, A., Rodda, B. E., Warrick, P., et. al. "Interactions of aspirin with nonsteroidal antiinflammatory drugs in man." Arth Rheum 19:4, 635-646, 1973.

Willkens, R. F. and Segre, E. J. "Combination therapy with naproxen and aspirin in rheumatoid arthritis." Arth Rheum 19:4, 677-682, 1976.

326. Q. Comment on the validity of the widely held view that intra-articular corticosteroid injections produce damage to the articular cartilage.

A. In a study of living adult human cartilage in tissue culture, critical assessment of hydrocortisone acetate in varying concentrations revealed no significant catabolic effect on the proteoglycan moiety. This study stands in contrast to other evidence from animal experiments demonstrating a depression of cartilage synthesis following intraarticular corticosteroids; morphological changes in the cartilage; decreased hexosamine content; and other similar changes. The issue has not yet been resolved. It has been suggested that perhaps the pain relief afforded in an arthritic joint by an intraarticular corticosteroid injection then allows greater use and increased weight-bearing eventually resulting in accelerated deterioration of the joint.

REF: Jacoby, R. K. "The effect of hydrocortisone acetate on adult human articular cartilage." J Rheum 3:4, 384-389, 1976.

327. Q. What effects on renal function does aspirin produce and of what clinical significance are these?

A. Significant but reversible effects on renal function may be seen with aspirin and other nonsteroidal antiinflammatory agents. Increases in serum creatinine and blood urea nitrogen levels have been described as well as decreased creatinine clearance rates up to 58% of normal. These changes were more apt to occur in patients with active renal disease. The clinical importance of these alterations in renal function is that monitoring of renal function may be affected and may lead to misinterpretations of clinical data.

REF: Kimberly, R. P. and Plotz, P. H. "Aspirin-induced depression of renal function." New Engl J Med 296:8, 418-424, 1977.

328. Q. Describe the effects of antiinflammatory drugs on lymphocytic response and comment on the clinical implications.

A. Various nonsteroidal antiinflammatory drugs including aspirin, as well as corticosteroids and penicillamine may affect various lymphocyte functions such as response to phytomitogen, antigenic stimulation, and mixed lymphocyte culture blastogenesis. These drugs include aspirin, phenylbutazone, indomethacin, sodium aurothiomalate, hydroxychloroquine, D-penicillamine, hydrocortisone, naproxen, and sodium melcofenamate. Combinations of drugs appeared to produce greater inhibition of lymphocyte responsiveness than did cultures of individual drugs. The clinical significance of these observations is that patients receiving these agents could have alterations in their cellular immunity, and additionally this could be one mechanism by which such agents could exert their antiinflammatory effect.

REF: Panush, R. S. "Effects of certain antirheumatic drugs on normal human peripheral blood lymphocytes." Arth Rheum 19:5, 907-917, 1976.

329. Q. Discuss the effectiveness, characteristics, and clinical indications of the propionic acid derivatives.

A. The propionic acid derivatives are all nonsteroidal antiinflammatory agents which include ibuprofen, naproxen, fenoprofen, and ketoprofen. They are all antipyretic and analgesic as well as being antiinflammatory. All are highly protein bound, inhibit prostaglandin synthesis, and in general exhibit less gastrointestinal toxicity and less gastrointestinal bleeding than salicylates. Naproxen and fenoprofen appear to be the most potent antiinflammatory agents in this group. These agents reach peak serum levels within 2 hours after ingestion and may be evaluated in terms of efficacy after 2 weeks of use. They have been given safely to patients with a history of peptic ulcer disease, giving them a distinct advantage over salicylates, indomethacin, and phenylbutazone.

REF: Huskisson, E. C. "Antiinflammatory drugs." Semin Arth Rheum 7:1, 1-20, 1977.

330. Q. What are the clinical characteristics of the newer nonsteroidal antiinflammatory agents that are not propionic acid derivatives but nonetheless resemble propionic acid derivatives clinically?

A. The drugs in this category are azopropazone, tolmetin, alclofenac, and the fenamates. Azopropazone is structurally similar to phenylbutazone but does not cause bone marrow toxicity. Its antiinflammatory potential is comparable to aspirin. Alclofenac has been compared to penicillamine in some studies, but skin rashes occur in 10% of patients and occasionally may be severe. Tolmetin is similar to indomethacin but with less gastrointestinal and central nervous system toxicity. Anthranilic acid derivatives are represented by mefenamic acid and flufenamic acid. They appear to possess greater gastrointestinal toxicity and diarrhea occurs in 15% of patients.

REF: Huskisson, E. C. "Antiinflammatory drugs." Semin Arth Rheum 7:1, 1-20, 1977.

331. Q. Discuss the hematologic toxicity of phenylbutazone.

A. This drug has its greatest usefulness in short term applications such as in the treatment of an acute attack of gout. Occasional patients with ankylosing spondylitis who do not benefit from various other nonsteroidal antiinflammatory agents should be treated with phenylbutazone. Bone marrow toxicity may take one of two forms. Granulocytopenia occurs in younger patients, is more common than aplastic anemia and tends to occur within the first month or two of treatment. Aplastic anemia is a more serious complication and carries a mortality rate of 50%. It tends to occur in elderly patients who have been treated for a year or more. The overall frequency of bone marrow toxic events is on the order of 1 in 66,000 prescriptions, making it a very rare event.   Nonetheless, phenylbutazone ranks as one of the leading causes of death in a report to the Committee on Safety of Medicines.

REF: Cuthbert, M. F. "Adverse reactions to nonsteroidal antirheumatic drugs." Curr Med Res Opin 2, 600-609, 1974.

Huskisson, E. C. "Antiinflammatory drugs." Semin Arth Rheum 7:1, 1-20, 1977.

332. Q.   What is the nature of gold induced hepatic injury?

A.   Gold rarely produces hepatic injury and hepatic toxicity resulting from gold remains unusual.   However, well defined hepatotoxicity has been noted with gold.   The features of this complication include elevation of the alkaline phosphatase, bilirubin, and LDH with the appearance of a cholestatic jaundice.   Liver biopsy reveals ballooning of the hepatocytes, bile stasis, and thrombi. Spontaneous recovery is the rule after gold is discontinued.

REF: Favreau, M. Tannenbauj, H. , and Lough, J. "Hepatic toxicity associated with gold therapy." Ann Intern Med 87, 717-719, 1977.

333. Q. Discuss tendon ruptures and their association with corticosteroids.

A.   Tendon ruptures have been associated with both systemic corticosteroids as well as local corticosteroid injections.   However, in many of these instances the etiological relationships are far from clear.   Frequently, the underlying disorder for which the steroids are being given is a collagen vascular disease itself capable of producing tendon rupture.   However, there is some experimental evidence that suggests a retardation of healing, decreased fibrosis, and decreased tensile strength of corticosteroids in the process of tendon repair.   The issue is further complicated by the observation that repetitive microruptures of tendons may present as "tendonitis" for which local corticosteroid injections could be given.

REF: Halpern, A.A. , Horowitz, B. G. , and Nagel, D. A. "Tendon ruptures associated with corticosteroid therapy." West J Med 127:5, 378-382, 1977.

334. Q. Discuss the theoretical and clinical basis for the use of colchicine in the treatment of familial Mediterranean fever, amyloidosis, and scleroderma.

A. Colchicine has been shown to block the synthesis of amyloid in animals in the casein model of amyloidogenesis. Inhibitory effects on leukocyte function have also been postulated. Colchicine has been implicated in collagen metabolism and has been demonstrated to disrupt microtubular function. It may increase collagenase activity and reduce the secretion of collagen precursors.

Because of these experimental and conceptual facts, colchicine was applied to the clinical treatment of various disorders associated with fibrosis. Preliminary clinical data suggest that familial Mediterranean fever may be amenable to treatment with colchicine as far as the acute attacks are concerned. Additionally, some evidence exists to suggest the possibility that amyloidosis and proteinuria may be responsive to treatment as well. However, despite an initial favorable report regarding the use of colchicine in scleroderma, more recent data has failed to confirm this finding.

Further investigation will be necessary before conclusions can be drawn regarding new uses for this old drug.

REF: Ravid, M., Robson, M., and Kedar (Keizman), I. "Prolonged colchicine treatment in four patients with amyloidosis." Ann Intern Med 87, 568-570, 1977.

Guttadauria, M., Diamond, H., and Kaplan, D. "Colchicine in the treatment of scleroderma." J Rheum 4:3, 272-276, 1977.

335. Q. Discuss the effect of D-penicillamine on serum and urine gold levels in patients treated initially with gold salts.

A. In the treatment of rheumatoid arthritis, gold and penicillamine both have antiinflammatory effects. However, penicillamine is also known to be a chelator of heavy metals. It has traditionally been advocated in the treatment of gold induced toxic events with the underlying assumption being that penicillamine chelates gold in vivo. However, in a study of 18 patients, serum and urinary gold levels did not appear to change significantly when patients were placed on pencillamine following an initial gold program. The speculative reasons why this should be so center on the high degree of protein binding of gold making the amount of free gold available for chelation relatively small.

REF: Davis, P., and Barraclough, D. "Interaction of D-penicillamine with gold salts." Arth Rheum 20:7, 1413-1418, 1977.

336. Q. "In a patient with rheumatoid arthritis on conventional chrysotherapy who does not seem to be responding to weekly injections of gold salts at 50 mgm, a trial of higher dose gold (75 mgm to 150 mgm) is warranted." Please comment on this statement in view of the current literature regarding gold salts.

A. The suggestion has been made in the literature that inadequate therapeutic responses to gold salts at the usual weekly dosage of 50 mgm may be due to inadequate serum levels of the drug. Therefore, measurement of serum gold levels with adjustment of the weekly dose of gold sometimes in excess of 50 mgm has been advocated. However, in a study of 47 patients, there was no correlation between serum gold levels and therapeutic response. Patients on conventional doses of gold (50 mgm weekly) did just as well as patients on high doses of gold (150 mgm weekly). However, complications of gold were significantly greater in the higher dose group. One could then conclude that the use of gold in higher weekly doses is not justified in a patient who does not respond to conventional doses of gold.

REF: Furst, D. E., Levine, S., Srinivasan, R., et. al. "A double blind trial of high versus conventional dosages of gold salts for rheumatoid salts." Arth Rheum 20:8, 1473-1480, 1977.

337. Q. Characterize the postinjection nonvasomotor reactions that can occur during chrysotherapy, estimate their frequency, and comment on their clinical significance.

A. Although once considered infrequent, nonvasomotor postinjection reactions have been noted in approximately 15% of patients. They include increased articular stiffness, myalgias, arthralgias, swelling, and constitutional symptoms. Their primary significance is that gold injections should not be prematurely terminated in such patients. Generally, substitution of gold thioglucose for sodium thiomalate will greatly ameliorate or abolish such reactions enabling continuation of the gold program.

REF: Halla, J. T., Hardin, J. G., and Linn, J. E. "Postinjection nonvasomotor reactions during chrysotherapy." Arth Rheum 20:6, 1188-1190, 1977.

338. Q. Compare the effect on prostaglandin synthesis of aspirin and various "aspirin-like" drugs in the nonsteroidal antiinflammatory category, and comment on the clinical significance.

A. Both aspirin and various aspirin-like drugs are potent inhibitors of prostaglandin synthesis. This fact has been used to consider this as possibly being significant in their antiinflammatory effects. Although the role of prostaglandins is not entirely clear, prostaglandins are known to increase vascular permeability and increase leukocyte migration. Furthermore, significant levels of prostaglandin E2 and prostaglandin F2 have been found in inflammatory exudates. Of interest is the observation that aspirin appears to inhibit prostaglandin synthesis in an irreversible manner as compared to aspirin-like drugs such as indomethacin, ibuprofen, and naproxen.

REF: Crook, D., Collins, A. J., Bacon, P. A., and Chan, R. "Prostaglandin synthetase activity from human rheumatoid synovial microsomes." Ann Rheum Dis 35, 327-332, 1976.

339. Q. Discuss the most frequent side effects that may be seen with cyclophosphamide in the treatment of rheumatic disorders.

A. Cyclophosphamide may produce hair loss, cystitis, azoospermia, anovulation, as well as gastrointestinal irritation, increased susceptibility to infections, teratogenesis, and possibly malignant disease.

REF: Decker, J. L. "Toxicity of immunosuppressive drugs in man." Arth Rheum 16:1, 89-91, 1973.

340. Q. What potential side effects and complications should you warn a patient about in whom you were considering the use of azathioprine?

A. Infectious complications, teratogenesis, possible hepatic damage, and the theoretical potential for neoplasia are the most worrisome features of azathioprine.

REF: Decker, J. L. "Toxicity of immunosuppressive drugs in man." Arth Rheum 16:1, 89-91, 1973.

341. Q. If methotrexate is given by intravenous or intramuscular injection, consider the potential side effects that could be encountered.

A. Oral ulcerations, gastrointestinal irritation, hair loss, increased infectious problems, teratogenesis, azoospermia, and possible hepatic damage are all noteworthy complications that have been reported in connection with methotrexate.

REF: Decker, J. L. "Toxicity of immunosuppressive drugs in man." Arth Rheum 16:1, 89-91, 1973.

342. Q. If you were asked to help draft a hospital protocol for the use of immunosuppressive and cytotoxic drugs in the treatment of rheumatic disorders, what important considerations would you give as guidelines for the use of these drugs?

A. In general the goals of therapy would be (a) to cure the disorder, if possible, (b) to suppress the manifestations of the disease, (c) to enable a reduction of an unacceptably high corticosteroid maintenance dosage, (d) to serve as an adjunctive medication to the concomitant use of other drugs, and (e) to prevent serious or life threatening complications of the underlying disease process. Certain requirements would have to be met such as the following: (1) the disease to be treated should be a life threatening or a seriously crippling disorder, (2) reversible clinical disease must be present, (3) a thorough trial of conventional, less toxic therapy must be given prior to considering these drugs, (4) there must be a diligent search for active infection, which should preclude the use of these drugs, (5) no underlying or potentially developing hematologic contraindication should be

present, (6) careful and comprehensive followup with objective measures of response should be instituted, (7) informed,
written consent should be obtained, (8) the protocol should
be submitted for peer review.

REF: Steinberg, A. D. "Efficacy of immunosuppressive
drugs in man." Arth Rheum 16:1, 92-96, 1973.

XIV. MISCELLANEOUS RHEUMATIC DISORDERS

343. Q. Describe the myopathy that has been noted in
Marfan's syndrome.

A. A slowly progressive myopathy has been described
with abnormal appearing mitochondria, concentric laminated
bodies on muscle microscopy, and abnormal densities of
uncertain significance.

REF: Goeble, K. M. , Muller, J. , DeMyer, W. "Myopathy
associated with Marfan's syndrome: fine structural and
histochemical observations." Neurology 23, 1257-1268,
1973.

344. Q. Discuss Dupuytren's contractures and comment on
treatment.

A. This process generally begins in the middle years
and often presents with small nodules at the distal palmar
area of one or both hands. The plantar fascia may also become involved early in the course of the disorder. Permanent contractures of one or several fingers occur. Fasciec-
tomy may be helpful. The triad of Dupuytren's contractures,
cataracts, and excessive alcoholic intake has been described.

REF: Vilijanto, J. A. "Dupuytren's contracture: a review".
Semin Arth Rheum 3, 155-176, 1974.

Sabiston, D. W. "Cataracts, Dupuytren's contracture, and
alcohol addiction." Am J Ophthalmol 76, 1005-1007, 1973.

345. Q. Catalogue the known causes of erythema nodosum.

A. In perhaps 25% of patients, no known cause exists.
However, the various causes that have been described include the following: (1) Infections, such as streptococcal,
tuberculosis, Yersinia, leprosy, herpes simplex, and many
others, (2) Sarcoidosis, (3) Inflammatory bowel disease,
(4) Drugs, such as sulfonamides, iodides, oral contra-
ceptives, (5) Behcet's disease, and (6) Pregnancy.

REF: Blomgren, S. E. "Erythema nodosum." Semin Arth
Rheum 4, 1-24, 1974.

346. Q. Describe erythema nodosum migrans.

A. The histology of erythema nodosum migrans is similar to that of erythema nodosum. The skin lesions are often unilateral and are far more chronic than in simple erythema nodosum. In most cases, these lesions persist for more than 9 months. The skin lesions are considered to be a variant of classical erythema nodosum and tend to spread centrifugally.

REF: Hannuksela, M. "Erythema nodosum migrans." Acta Derm Venereol 53, 313-317, 1973.

347. Q. Describe the clinical features of the arthritis of sickle cell anemia.

A. When arthritis occurs in sickle cell anemia, it is generally in the context of a sickle cell crisis, and not the presenting symptom. A migratory, polyarticular pattern is the rule and monoarticular disease rarely noted. In children, a propensity for hand and foot involvement is noted.

REF: Espinoza, L.R., Spilberg, I., and Osterland, C.K. "Joint manifestations of sickle cell disease." Medicine 53, 295-305, 1974.

348. Q. What would one expect to find in the synovial fluid analysis of a sickle cell-associated acute arthritis? Also, comment on the histological features of the synovium.

A. The synovial fluid is generally of a noninflammatory kind. Although occasionally polymorphonuclear cells may predominate, in general the most commonly seen cell is the mononuclear cell. In half of the patients, one may see sickled red blood cells. Histologically, the synovium reveals little inflammatory changes and sickled cells may be seen within blood vessels, many of which are thrombosed. Hypertrophy of the focal lining cells is seen.

REF: Schumacher, H.R., Andrews, R., and McLaughlin, G. "Arthropathy in sickle cell disease." Ann Intern Med 78, 203-211, 1973.

Espinoza, L.R., Spilberg, I., and Osterland, M.K. "Joint manifestations of sickle cell disease." Medicine 53, 295-305, 1974.

349. Q. Describe the structure and immunochemistry of amyloid deposits.

A. Amyloid occurs in fibrils of 40 to 60 A in diameter. Two proteins constitute these fibrils. The AL protein is a portion of the amino terminal segment of a light chain derived from an immunoglobulin and is present in primary amyloidosis and amyloid associated with myeloma. The AA protein is a non immunoglobulin protein which forms the major component in secondary amyloid deposits and in familial amyloidosis. An entirely separate protein component found in amyloid deposits is P component and may be related to the first component of complement.

REF: Scheinberg, M.A. "Immunology of amyloid disease: A review." Semin Arth Rheum 7:2, 133-140, 1977.

350. Q. What is SAA protein and what is its significance in amyloidosis?

A. SAA protein appears to be a precursor of AA protein and can be found in the serum of patients with amyloidosis of both the primary and secondary type. Although it can be found in cord blood in small concentrations, its level in the serum increases with age. There is accumulating evidence that SAA may be present in a wide variety of disorders, both infectious and rheumatic. It may bear correlation with disease activity in such rheumatic disorders as juvenile rheumatoid arthritis.

REF: Scheinberg, M.A. "Immunology of amyloid disease: A review." Semin Arth Rheum 7:2, 133-140, 1977.

351. Q. Discuss the frequency of M components in primary and secondary amyloidosis.

A. Although some controversy exists regarding this question, in general it is believed that evidence of a monoclonal gammopathy (M components) exists in primary amyloidosis and in amyloidosis associated with multiple myeloma. However, in patients who have secondary forms of amyloidosis and hereditofamilial forms, the serum and urine remains generally free of M components.

REF: Scheinberg, M.A. and Cathcart, E.S. "Comprehensive study of humoral and cellular immune abnormalities in 26 patients with systemic amyloidosis." Arth Rheum 19:173, 1976.

352. Q. Comment on the role of radionuclide joint imaging in the rheumatic diseases.

A. At the present time the most useful area for radionuclide joint imaging is in the patient with arthralgias but without objective clinical signs. In such patients, joint scanning has demonstrated greater sensitivity than can otherwise be obtained by conventional radiographs and clinical assessment of articular swelling. It can also be used in the assessment of subclinical areas of joint involvement in patients with well established disease and in following patients on treatment.

REF: Rosenthall, L., and Hawkins, D. "Radionuclide joint imaging in the diagnosis of synovial disease." Semin Arth Rheum 7:1, 49-61, 1977.

353. Q. Discuss the varying nature of the subcutaneous nodule in rheumatic disorders.

A. The rheumatoid nodule is the most commonly seen subcutaneous nodule and consists of a central zone of necrosis, a second layer of palisading histiocytic cells, surrounded by fibrosis. The rheumatoid nodule is of long duration and correlates with severity of disease. In contrast, the rheumatic nodule is short lived and does not correlate with arthritic involvement, but does correlate with cardiac involvement. The nodules of juvenile rheumatoid arthritis appear to be histologically similar to those of rheumatic fever. Rheumatoid variant disorders, systemic lupus erythematosus, Behcet's syndrome, are other disorders in which subcutaneous nodules may be seen.

REF: Niirem, C.P. and Willkens, R.F. "The subcutaneous nodule: its significance in the diagnosis of rheumatic disease." Semin Arth Rheum 7:1, 63-79, 1977.

354. Q. What are the clinical features of gram-negative septic arthritis?

A. Patients who are elderly, who have serious systemic disease, who are on immunosuppressive durgs, and who are drug addicts are predisposed to develop gram negative septic arthritis. However, some patients appear to develop this problem without apparent underlying factors. An associated osteomyelitis may be present. The onset is usually insidious and fever with chills may be absent. Pseudomonas aeruginosa is the usual infecting organism in 50% of cases.

REF: Bayer, A.S., Chow, A.W., Louie, J.S., et.al. "Gram negative bacillary septic arthritis: clinical, radiographic, therapeutic, and prognostic features." Semin Arth Rheum 7:2, 123-132, 1977.

355. Q. Discuss the diagnostic procedures necessary in gram negative septic arthritis and comment on treatment.

A. The radiographs of involved joints generally reveal evidence of erosions and periosteal elevation. Needle aspiration may fail to yield positive cultures, and open arthrotomy with appropriate cultures and debridement appears necessary in most cases. Treatment is therefore both surgical and medical, the latter being guided by specific bacterial sensitivity studies.

REF: Bayer, A.S., Chow, A.W., Louie, J.S., et.al. "Gram negative bacillary septic arthritis: clinical, radiographic, therapeutic, and prognostic features." Semin Arth Rheum 7:2, 123-132, 1977.

356. Q. What is the expected prognosis in a patient with gram negative septic arthritis and associated osteomyelitis?

A. In contrast to earlier studies, more recent data suggest that in a patient treated with a combination of surgical and medical modalities with antibiotics chosen by appropriate sensitivity testing, the general result is favorable. Only 10% of patients develop residual functional impairment.

Stabilization and healing of radiographic lesions is the rule. Chronic or recurrent infection is usually absent.

REF: Bayer, A.S., Chow, A.W., Louie, J.S., et.al. "Gram negative bacillary septic arthritis: clinical, radiographic, therapeutic, and prognostic features." Semin Arth Rheum 7:2, 123-132, 1977.

357. Q. Discuss the immunology of recurrent bacteriuria.

A. There is increasing evidence to suggest that cervicovaginal antibody is important in the pathogenesis of recurrent bacteriuria. IgA and IgG are the most commonly seen antibodies, but IgM is also present. In patients who are susceptible to recurrent bacteriuria, cervicovaginal antibodies are present in 26% of patients, whereas in patients resistant to recurrent bacteriuria, 77% had adequate antibody to Enterobacteriaceae.

REF: Stamey, T.A., Wehner, N., Milhara, G., and Condy, M. "The immunological basis of recurrent bacteriuria: Role of cervicovaginal antibody in Enterobacterial colonization of the introital mucosa." Medicine 57:1, 47-56, 1977.

358. Q. What initial disorder is felt to be instrumental in the development of adhesive capsulitis and the frozen shoulder syndrome?

A. Although areas of controversy exist among orthopedic surgeons and rheumatologists, tendinitis of the supraspinatus tendon is felt by many to be the initial step in the development of the frozen shoulder syndrome and adhesive capsulitis of the shoulder.

REF: Bland, J.H., Merrit, J.A., and Boushey, D.R. "The painful shoulder." Semin Arth Rheum 7:1, 21-47, 1977.

359. Q. Describe the proposed steps in the evolution of a frozen shoulder from an uncomplicated "painful shoulder."

A. In general it is felt that tendinitis of the supraspinatus tendon leads to spread of the inflammation in the tendon sheath with eventual rupture into the subacromial bursa.

The inflammation then becomes more generalized extending into the humeral head as osteitis. A "frozen shoulder" may develop when there is widespread inflammation involving the tendons, bursa, capsule, synovium, muscle, and other supporting structures. Fibrous tissue leads to soft tissue contracture and diminished volume of the shoulder joint.

REF: Bland, J.H., Merrit, J.A., and Boushey, D.R. "The painful shoulder." Semin Arth Rheum 7:1, 21-47, 1977.

360. Q. Discuss the signs and symptoms of reflex sympathetic dystrophy syndrome.

A. In general the most common symptoms of this syndrome are pain and swelling of the affected extremity. Various trophic changes occur including cyanosis, the development of a shiny skin overlying the involved area, generalized edema, skin tenderness, hypertrichosis and hyperhidrosis, hypertrophic nails, and loss of bony landmarks. Vasomotor abnormalities such as hyperesthesia, vasospasm, and vasodilatation are noted. Functional impairment is generally extensive. Pain, diffuse tenderness, restricted mobility in all ranges of motion and aching are characteristic.

REF: Bland, J.H., Merrit, J.A., and Boushey, D.R. "The painful shoulder." Semin Arth Rheum 7:1, 21-47, 1977.

361. Q. Discuss the most common areas of nerve entrapment syndromes in the upper extremity for the median nerve.

A. Although the carpal tunnel syndrome at the wrist is perhaps the best known type of entrapment syndrome for the median nerve, there are other sites where the median nerve may be compressed giving rise to clinial symptoms. These additional areas include: (1) the supracondylar area above the elbow, the proximal forearm at the pronator muscle, the anterior interosseous in the forearm, and digital compression in the hand.

REF: Cracchiolo, A., III, Namerow, N.S., Campion, D.S. et. al. "Peripheral nerve entrapments." West J Med 127, 299-313, 1977.

362. Q. What are the most commonly seen sites of ulnar nerve entrapment?

A. Ulnar nerve compression may occur at the thoracic outlet, at the elbow in the cubital tunnel, and in the hand. The latter includes the proximal and distal Guyon's tunnel, and the digital areas.

REF: Cracchiolo, A., III, Namerow, N.S., Campion, D.S. et.al. "Peripheral nerve entrapments." West J Med 127, 299-313, 1977.

363. Q. Name the sites of radial nerve entrapment in the upper extremity.

A. The sites of compression of the radial nerve are at the axilla, at the humerus ("Saturday night palsy"), and in the forearm. The muscles which cause the latter compression are the supinator, posterior interosseous, and the superficial cutaneous.

REF: Cracchiolo, A., III, Namerow, N.S., Campion, D.S., et.al. "Peripheral nerve entrapments." West J Med 127, 299-313, 1977.

364. Q. What is the sequence of electromyographic abnormalities that one would expect to find in the carpal tunnel syndrome with increasing severity of involvement and compression of the median nerve?

A. The earliest electromyographic changes seen in early and mild carpal tunnel syndrome are decreases in the potential amplitude of sensory nerve stimulation. Sensory latency may be prolonged. As moderate degrees of compression are encountered, then motor potential is decreased and motor latency is prolonged. Finally, conduction velocity will decrease toward moderately severe levels of compression. When denervation potentials are found, then compression is felt to have reached the severe stage.

REF: Cracchiolo, A., III, Namerow, N.S., Campion, D.S. et.al. "Peripheral nerve entrapments." West J Med 127, 299-313, 1977.

365. Q. Review the factors which are important in the development of various peripheral nerve compression syndromes.

A. The most important pathogenetic factors in peripheral nerve compression are these: (1) Superficial and therefore susceptible nerve location. The ulnar nerve at the elbow, the radial nerve at the axialla, the peroneal nerve at the knee are all examples of this type of vulnerability. (2) Potentially confined peripheral nerves such as the median nerve at the wrist, the ulnar nerve at the wrist, the deep radial nerve at the elbow, and the tarsal nerve at the ankle. (3) Swollen or enlarged peripheral nerves such as in hypothyroidism, acromegaly, familial amyloidosis, hypertrophic neuropathy, and leprosy.

REF: Cracchiolo, A., III, Namerow, N.S., Campion, D.S. et. al. "Peripheral nerve entrapments." West J Med 127, 299-313, 1977.

366. Q. In postmenopausal women, does the addition of calcium carbonate and the use of estrogens improve osteoporosis and decrease bone turnover?

A. In a study of 60 postmenopausal women, careful evaluation disclosed that the use of estrogen products appeared to decrease bone loss by suppressing bone turnover rates. Resorption was decreased more than bone accretion, with the net effect that bone loss was diminished. Calcium supplementation also appeared to produce similar beneficial effects. Although the issue is still controversial and further data are needed, the authors concluded that the use of estrogen and calcium supplementation would be likely to halt further bone loss in the osteoporotic postmenopausal women.

REF: Recker, R.R., Saville, P.D., and Heaney, R.P. "Effect of estrogens and calcium carbonate on bone loss in postmenopausal women." Ann Intern Med 87, 649-655, 1977.

367. Q. Any attempt to name the most significant contributions to American Rheumatology will certainly be a subjective undertaking, and no "right" or "wrong" answer is

possible. However, with these limitations in mind, what are the 12 most significant and important contributions to the understanding of rheumatic disease, in your opinion ?

A. In his presidential address to the American Rheumatism Association, Dr. Gerald P. Rodnan quoted the following list. (1) The discovery of the rheumatoid factor and the subsequent description of the role of antiglobulins in the inflammatory rheumatoid response. (2) The lupus cell preparation. (3) The clinical introduction of corticosteroid medication. (4) Immune complex mediated disease and systemic lupus erythematosus. (5) Gout, pseudogout, and the concept of crystal induced synovitis. (6) Hyperuricemia due to enzymatic defects and overproduction of uric acid in certain types of gout. (7) Probenecid. (8) Allopurinol. (9) Spondyloarthritic disorders and the association of the HLA-B27 antigen. (10) The streptococcus in the pathogenesis of rheumatic fever. (11) Chemoprophylaxis of rheumatic fever. (12) Specific defects in enzymes in the heritable disorders of connective tissue.

REF: Rodnan, G. P. "Growth and development of rheumatology in the United States.   A bicentennial report." Arth Rheum 20:6, 1149-1168, 1977.

368. Q. As a practicing rheumatologist in private practice, what are the most common rheumatological problems that you are likely to encounter ?

A. The most commonly seen rheumatological problem is some type of musculoskeletal "soft tissue" disorder such as bursitis, tendinitis,fibrositis, and so forth. Low back syndromes are next in frequency, followed by rheumatoid arthritis, and then degenerative osteoarthritis. Connective tissue disorders, such as systemic lupus erythematosus, scleroderma, and others, were far less commonly seen.

REF: The American Rheumatism Association Committee on Rheumatology Practice. "A description of rheumatology practice." Arth Rheum 20:6, 1278-1281, 1977.

369. Q. What are the features of papular mucinosis?

A. Papular mucinosis is an unusual disorder of mucopolysaccharide deposition presenting with cutaneous manifestations and a characteristic IgG lambda light chain paraproteinemia. Although the disorder has generally been felt to be a relatively benign chronic disease, it has also been associated with arthritis, myopathy and eosinophilia.

REF: McAdam, L.P., Pearson, C.M., Pitts, W.H., et.al. Arth Rheum 20:4, 989-996, 1977.

370. Q. Discuss the musculoskeletal manifestations of bacterial endocarditis.

A. A large number of patients with bacterial endo-carditis may develop musculoskeletal complaints. In one series of 192 cases, the frequency of musculoskeletal symp-toms was 44%. Arthralgias and arthritis were the most commonly seen. Diffuse myalgias were also noted. These were often unilateral and asymmetrical. Monoarticular or oligoarticular arthritis was the rule. That musculoskeletal manifestations were the presenting feature in perhaps 27% of cases attests to the importance in recognizing this complication in bacterial endocarditis.

REF: Churchill, M.A., Geraci, J.E., Hunder, G.G. "Musculoskeletal manifestations of bacterial endocarditis." Ann Intern Med 87:754-759, 1977.

371. Q. Compare the frequency of arthritic complications in chronic ulcerative colitis and Crohn's disease.

A. In general, it has been estimated that arthritis occurs in perhaps 23% of patients with inflammatory bowel disease. Patients with colonic involvement (27%) appear to have more frequent arthritis than patients with small bowel disease (14%). In Crohn's disease limited to the colon, the incidence of arthritis was 39%.

REF: Greenstein, A.J., Janowitz, H.D., and Sachar, D.B. "The extraintestinal complications of Crohn's disease and ulcerative colitis: A study of 700 patients." Medicine 55:4, 401-412, 1976.

372. Q. What are the various types of arthritis that may be seen in inflammatory bowel disease, and comment on the

association of these different types of arthritis with the
HLA-B27 antigen?

A.   Peripheral joint disease is typically inflammatory,
non-deforming and non-erosive. Large joints such as the
knees are most typically affected. There is little or no correlation between peripheral joint disease and the B27 antigen.
This type of arthritis appears to follow the course of the inflammatory bowel symptoms. Involvement of the sacroiliac
joints and the spine may occur and mimic ankylosing spondylitis. This type of arthritis is independent of the clinical
course of the inflammatory bowel disease, and it is correlated
with the HLA-B27 antigen in perhaps 50% of cases.

REF: Greenstein, A.J., Janowitz, H.D., and Sachar, D.B.
"The extraintestinal complications of Crohn's disease and
ulcerative colitis: A study of 700 patients." Medicine 55:4,
401-412, 1976.

Kemple, K. and Bluestone, R. "The histocompatibility complex and rheumatic diseases." Med Clin North Am, 61:2,
331-345, March 1977

373. Q. Discuss the type of arthritis seen after intestinal
bypass surgery for intractable obesity.

A.   The arthritis most commonly seen is that of large
joint involvement. Initially, arthritis was felt to be a pecu-
liar manifestation of jejunocolostomy procedures. However,
more recently it has become clear that jejunoilesotomy procedures may also be associated with arthritis of a similar
kind. Although the sedimentation rate may be elevated, it
need not be so in all cases. Treatment with nonsteroidal
antiinflammatory agents is helpful. Surgical removal of the
bypass procedure generally results in improvement in the
arthritic symptoms.

REF: Fernandez Herlihy, L. "Arthritis after jejunoileos-
tomy for intractable obesity." J Rheum 4:2, 135-138, 1977.

374. Q. Discuss the causes of protrusio acetabuli.

A.   A common type of protrusio is the developmental
form beginning in childhood upon which superimposed degenerative changes may occur. Inflammatory disorders

such as rheumatoid arthritis, ankylosing spondylitis, juvenile rheumatoid arthritis, and others may produce this complication. Septic arthritis, Paget's disease, rickets, osteomalacia, fractures, Charcot joint disease, metastatic disease, and pelvic irradiation, are other causes.

REF: Hasselbacher, P. and Schumacher, H. R. "Bilateral protrusio acetabuli following pelvic irradiation." J Rheum 4:2, 189-196, 1977.

375. Q. What is the syndrome of transient osteoporosis of the hip?

A. This is a painful, self limited condition of unknown cause which generally lasts less than one year with full recovery. The only roentgenological manifestation is localized osteoporosis. Men and women are affected with trauma and pregnancy being related factors. The sedimentation rate and serological studies are typically normal.

REF: Valenzuela, F., Aris, H., and Jacobelli, S. "Transient osteoporosis of the hip." J Rheum 4:1, 59-64, 1977.

376. Q. Discuss alkaptonuria and the musculoskeletal manifestations that are usually seen in this disorder.

A. The lumbar spine is the first area to become involved in ochronosis, usually in the third decade. Involvement of the intervertebral discs, brittleness, calcification, intervertebral osteophytic bridging, and fusion of the vertebral bodies are not infrequent manifestations. Peripheral joint involvement usually occurs later in the disease, perhaps some 10 years or so after the spinal manifestations. Recurrent synovitis and joint effusions, sometimes simulating rheumatoid arthritis, may be observed.

REF: Lagier, R. and Sitaj, S. "Vertebral changes in ochronosis, anatomical and radiological study of one case." Ann Rheum Dis 33, 86-92, 1974.

377. Q. Describe the clinical and radiographic changes noted in diabetic arthropathy.

A. The most commonly observed features of diabetic neuropathic arthropathy include: (1) articular swelling,

(2) subluxation, (3) fracture and progressive fragmentation, (4) subchondral osteoporosis, (5) bony sclerosis in adjacent bone.

REF: Clouse, M. E., Gramm, H. F., Legg, M., et. al. "Diabetic osteoarthropathy: Clinical and roentgenographic observations in 90 cases. Am J Roentgenol Radium Ther Nucl Med 121, 22-34, 1974.

378. Q. In children born with deformities of the limbs resulting from thalidomide, what are the typical radiographic changes seen in the joints of these unfortunate children?

A. The radiographic picture of thalidomide-induced deformities is quite similar to that which has been described in classical neuropathic joint disease. Extensive and often bizarre osteophytosis, fragmentation and trabecular disorganization, sclerosis, osseous fragmentation, cartilaginous and bony debri, and rapid distortion of the joint architecture are all typical features.

REF: McCredie, J. "Thalidomide and congenital Charcot's joints." Lancet, 2, 1058-1061, 1973.

379. Q. What is Behcet's syndrome and how does it generally present clinically?

A. The following triad has clasically defined Behcet's syndrome: (1) oral ulcerations, (2) genital ulcerations, and (3) ocular lesions. In general, the presenting symptoms of Behcet's syndrome are one or several of these components. However, it has become increasingly evident that Behcet's syndrome represents a widespread and systemic disorder which may involve multiple organ systems leading to diverse symptoms.

REF: Chajek, T., Fainaru, M. "Behcet's disease. Report of 41 cases and a review of the literature." Medicine 54, 179-196, 1975.

380. Q. Describe the many multisystemic features of Behcet's syndrome that may be seen in addition to the classical "triad" that defines this disease.

A. Many organ systems may be affected by Behcet's syndrome. Therefore, a wide variety of symptoms may be seen. These include thrombophlebitis, aseptic meningitis, central nervous system involvement, colitis, pulmonary lesions, benign intracranial hypertension, recurrent Bell's palsy, thrombotic venous and arterial lesions, vena cava syndrome, vasculitis, and arthritis.

REF: Chajek, T., Aronowski, E., and Izak, G. "Decreased fibrinolysis in Behcet's disease." Thromb Diath Haemorrh 29, 610-618, 1973.

Chajek, T., Fainaru, M. "Behcet's disease. Report of 41 cases and a review of the literature." Medicine, 54, 179-196, 1975.

381. Q. What tumors might cause diagnostic confusion in rheumatic disorders such as rheumatoid arthritis?

A. Several tumors must be kept in mind by the rheumatologist because in rare instances they may mimic inflammatory arthritis such as rheumatoid arthritis. The tumors which are most likely to cause diagnostic confusion are pigmented villonodular synovitis, benign and malignant synovial chondrometaplasia, chondrosarcoma, synovial sarcoma, and osteoid osteoma.

REF: Twenty Second Rheumatism Review. Tumors. Arth Rheum 19:6 (Supplement), 1094-1095, 1976.

382. Q. Discuss the syndrome of malignant hyperpyrexia myopathy.

A. This is an often fatal complication of general anesthesia, frequently halothane. The basis of the disorder appears to be an inherent abnormality of muscle metabolism such that when an appropriate triggering mechanism occurs, there is a very rapid and excessive muscle contraction with the production of excessive heat. Familial aggregation has been noted, and subclinical elevation of the CPK has occasionally identified individuals at risk.

REF: Harriman, D.G.F., Summer, D.W., and Ellis, F.R. "Malignant hyperpyrexia myopathy." Q J Med 42, 639-658, 1973.

383. Q. Discuss the incidence of rheumatic fever in the United States and some of the epidemiological factors of most significance.

A. In school children followed with serial throat cultures, hemolytic streptococcal infections were noted in approximately 18% of all throat cultures of which 11% were group A streptococci. The most important factor was socioeconomic status in that twice the frequency of streptococcal infection was noted in lower socioeconomic groups as compared to children in middle or higher socioeconomic groups. Rheumatic fever was more prevalent among blacks than among whites, and was most frequent in the 5- to 19-year-old group. The highest incidence of rheumatic fever occurred in 10- to 14-year old blacks where a figure of 55.5 cases per 100,000 children was noted. In Manhattan the case rate was 61 and in Baltimore 10.6 cases per 100,000. Although considered to be an area of infrequently seen rheumatic fever, Miami reported 95 patients with rheumatic fever, reminding one that the disease is still found throughout the United States.

REF: Quinn, R.W., and Federspeil, C. F. "The incidence of rheumatic fever in metropolitan Nashville, 1963 to 1969." Am J Epidemiol 99, 273-280, 1973.

Brownell, K.D., and Bailen Rose, F. "Acute rheumatic fever in children. Incidence in a borough of New York City." JAMA 224, 1593-1597, 1973.

384. Q. Describe the streptozyme test and comment on its usefulness in the diagnosis of rheumatic fever and streptococcal infections.

A. The streptozyme test was introduced in 1971 and involves a simple slide agglutination of sensitized sheep erythrocytes. Its usefulness is in presenting multiple streptococcal antigens and thereby increasing the sensitivity of screening for streptococcal infections. In general, the streptozyme test becomes positive in 6 to 9 days following infections with streptococcal organisms and will detect such infections in 73 to 95% of individuals.

REF: Bisno, A.L. and Ofek, I. "Serologic diagnosis of streptococcal infection: Comparison of a rapid

hemagglutination technique with conventional antibody tests."
Am J Dis Child 127, 676-681, 1974.

385. Q. Discuss the inherited disorders of connective
tissue.

A. Six disorders have been characterized. These include: (1) Hurler syndrome, clouding of the cornea, grave manifestations, (2) Hunter syndrome, without corneal clouding and a milder course, (3) Sanfilippo syndrome, with severe CNS effects, (4) Morquio syndrome with severe bony changes, corneal clouding, intellectual impairment and aortic insufficiency, (5) Scheie syndrome, stiff joints, corneal clouding, impairment of intellect, and aortic insufficiency, and (6) Maroteaux-Lamy syndrome with extensive osseous and corneal changes. They are all inherited as autosomal recessives except for Hunter's syndrome (Type II), which is inherited as an x-linked recessive.

REF: Beighton, P. "The inherited disorders of connective tissue." Bull Rheum Dis 23:3, 702-707, 1972-73.

386. Q. What is fibrodysplasia ossificans progressiva?

A. This is a rare disorder involving recurrent episodes of inflammation in the tendons, fascia, and soft tissues resulting in eventual ossification at these sites. Microdactyly may accompany this disorder which produces no systemic manifestations, but generally progresses to incapacitating generalized rigidity.

REF: Beighton, P. "The inherited disorders of connective tissue." Bull Rheum Dis 23:3, 702-707, 1972-73.

387. Q. Describe Leri's pleonosteosis.

A. This is a rare disorder of unknown cause wherein fibrous hyperplasia of the joint capsules and ligaments produces broad digits, flexion deformities, and decreased mobility of the hands and feet. Carpal tunnel syndrome and metatarsalgia may occur. It is inherited as an autosomal dominant trait.

REF: Beighton, P. "The inherited disorders of connective tissue." Bull Rheum Dis 23:3, 702-707, 1972-73.

388. Q. What is osteopoikilosis and what is its significance?

A. This is generally a radiographic diagnosis of no particular clinical significance other than to differentiate it from bony malignant metastases. Disrete areas of sclerosis in bones are noted, often near the hip joints.

REF: Beighton, P. "The inherited disorders of connective tissue." Bull Rheum Dis 23:3, 702-707, 1972-73.

389. Q. Discuss cutis laxa.

A. Extreme laxity of the skin occurs as an inherited disorder such that the appearance of old age may occur even in childhood. No joint changes occur, the joints are not lax, and the skin is not unduly fragile, features which distinguish this disorder from Ehlers-Danlos syndrome.

REF: Beighton, P. "The inherited disorders of connective tissue." Bull Rheum Dis, 23:3, 702-707, 1972-73.

390. Q. What are the features of reticulohistiocytosis?

A. Diffuse xanthomatous giant cell granulomatous lesions develop in the skin, mucous membranes, and synovial membranes. Xanthelasma may be seen, and women are affected more frequently than men. Erosive and destructive polyarthritis may occur involving any joint, but particularly the hands.

REF: Boyle, J.A. and Buchanan, W.W. "Clinical Rheumatology." Blackwell Scientific Publications, Oxford and Edinburgh. 1971, 407-409.

391. Q. What is benign intermittent hydrarthrosis?

A. This is a recurrent episodic inflammatory arthritis of joints, particularly of the knees, which occurs in females shortly following puberty. The condition is characterized by a regularity of symptoms, the interval between attacks being relatively constant for any given individual.

REF: Boyle, J.A. and Buchanan, W.W. "Clinical Rheumatology." Blackwell Scientific Publications, Oxford and Edinburgh. 1971, 409-410.

392. Q. Discuss palindromic rheumatism and its possible relationship to rheumatoid arthritis.

A. This is a condition of sudden pain, swelling, and inflammatory changes in one or several joints, usually lasting less than a week. Increasing evidence suggests that this may be a form of early seronegative rheumatoid arthritis. Patients followed for long periods of time with this diagnosis generally develop clinical and radiographic changes consistent with rheumatoid disease.

REF: Boyle, J.A. and Buchanan, W.W. "Clinical Rheumatology." Blackwell Scientific Publications, Oxford and Edinburgh, 1971, 410.

393. Q. Discuss the "stiff-man syndrome."

A. Symmetrical stiffness of the muscles usually occurs in the fifth decade. Both men and women are affected. The proximal and truncal muscles are more commonly involved than are the distal muscles. The facial muscles are uninvolved. The diagnosis is facilitated by electromyographic evidence of continuous firing of muscle fibers with potentials that resemble voluntary muscle contractions. There is no electrical silence in involved muscles. Serum enzymes and muscle biopsy remain normal. Treatment is generally with diazepam.

REF: Boyle, J.A. and Buchanan, W.W. "Clinical Rheumatology." Blackwell Scientific Publications, Oxford and Edinburgh, 1971, 436.

394. Q. Describe the typical "march fracture" or Deutschlander's disease.

A. This is generally a stress fracture of the second or third metatarsal and occurs as a result of excessive walking or marching. Localized pain and tenderness is noted at the area of the fracture and edema may occur on the dorsum of the involved foot. In the early stages, the radiographs may be normal, although in two or three weeks, a typical fracture pattern may be noted. Treatment is with rest and splinting.

REF: Boyle, J.A. and Buchanan, W.W. "Clinical Rheumatology." Blackwell Scientific Publications, Oxford and Edinburgh, 1971, 442.

395. Q. What are the usual symptoms and radiographic appearance of osteochondritis of the metatarsal head (Freiberg's or Kohler's disease)?

A. There is pain and tenderness at the head of the second metatarsal with localized swelling. X-rays reveal flattening of the head of the involved metatarsal with irregularity of the borders.

REF: Boyle, J.A. and Buchanan, W.W. "Clinical Rheumatology." Blackwell Scientific Publications, Oxford and Edinburgh, 1971, 442-443.

396. Q. What are the serological findings typical of mixed connective tissue disease?

A. The disease is defined by the presence of extractable nuclear antigen containing ribonuclease sensitive ribonucleoprotein. In general, the antinuclear antibody titer is positive and of the speckled pattern.

REF: Sharp, G.C., Irvin, W.S., May, C.M., et.al. "Association of antibodies to ribonucleoprotein and Sm antigens with mixed connective tissue disease, systemic lupus erythematosus and other rheumatic diseases." New Engl J Med 295:21, 1149-1154, 1976.

397. Q. What are the usual clinical features of mixed connective tissue disease?

A. Raynaud's phenomenon, swollen hands, myositis, arthritis or arthralgias, decreased esophageal motility, and sclerodermatous skin changes constitute the most common clinical features of mixed connective tissue disease. Other features generally include fever, serositis, decreased pulmonary diffusing capacity, lymphadenopathy, hepatomegaly and splenomegaly. Significant renal disease is usually absent. The syndrome responds to corticosteroid medication, and the course is benign.

REF: Sharp, G. C., Irvin, W. S., May, C. M., et. al. "Association of antibodies to ribonucleoprotein and Sm antigen with mixed connective tissue disease, systemic lupus erythematosus, and other rheumatic diseases." New Engl J Med 295:21, 1149-1154, 1976.

398. Q. Which rheumatic disorders most often resemble the clinical features found in mixed connective tissue disease?

A. Perhaps the most difficult diagnostic distinction to draw is between mixed connective tissue disease and systemic lupus erythematosus. Other rheumatic diseases which may also cause confusion are scleroderma, polymyositis, and rheumatoid arthritis.

REF: Leibfarth, J. H. and Persellin, R. H. "Characteristics of patients with serum antibodies to extractable nuclear antigens." Arth and Rheum 19:5, 851-856, 1976.

399. Q. Characterize the lymphocytotoxic antibodies that are found in mixed connective tissue disease.

A. These are generally of the IgG or IgM class and are cold reactive. Their immunochemical characteristics are similar to those found in systemic lupus erythematosus. The antibodies belonging to the IgM class are more cytotoxic for lymphocytes than are the antibodies belonging to the IgG class. In one study, 59% of sera tested from patients with mixed connective tissue disease were positive for cold-reactive lymphocytotoxic antibodies.

REF: Diaz Jouanen, E., Llorente, L., Ramos Niembro, F., and Alarcon Segovia, D. "Cold reactive lymphocytotoxic antibodies in mixed connective tissue disease." J Rheum 4:1, 4-10, 1977.

400. Q. Characterize the aseptic necrosis seen in renal transplantation patients.

A. Aseptic necrosis of bone is not rare in renal transplantation. Multiple sites are present in 85% of patients.

The onset of aseptic necrosis begins generally within the first 1 to 2 years after transplantation. Osteoporosis and hyperparathyroid bone disease appear to be correlated.

REF: Ibels, L. S., Alfrey, A. C., Huffer, W. E., and Weil, R., III. "Aseptic necrosis of bone following renal transplantation: Experience in 194 transplant recipients and review of the literature." Medicine, 57:1, 25-45, 1977.

401. Q. Discuss the relationship of aseptic bone necrosis in renal transplant patients to corticosteroid administration and comment on the possible mechanisms by which this effect might occur.

A. Although the role of steroid medication has not yet been clearly defined in this situation, it is nonetheless probable that corticosteroids are related to the pathogenesis of aseptic bone necrosis. When prednisone is decreased to less than 100 mgm daily during the first month following transplantation, the frequency of aseptic necrosis of bone appears to diminish. The mechanisms by which aseptic necrosis of bone might occur are as follows: (1) Ischemic bone necrosis could occur if corticosteroid medication induced a hyperlipidemic state, along with a fatty liver, and peripheral systemic fat embolization. (2) Another theoretical model of bone necrosis would relate the hyperparathyroidism noted in uremic transplantation patients to osteoporosis induced by corticosteroid medication with subsequent microfractures with weight bearing.

REF: Ibels, L. S., Alfrey, A. C., Huffer, W. E., and Weil, R., III. "Aseptic necrosis of bone following renal transplantation: Experience in 194 transplant recipients and review of the literature." Medicine, 57:1, 25-45, 1977.

402. Q. Discuss the factors which are most helpful in the diagnosis of the "fibrositis" syndrome.

A. Patients with the "fibrositis" syndrome frequently complain of chronic aching, marked morning stiffness and fatigue, localized tenderness in specific and characteristic musculoskeletal sites, and certain electroencephalographic findings.

REF: Smythe, H.A. and Moldofsky, H. "Two contributions to understanding of the "fibrositis" syndrome." Bull Rheum Dis 28:1, 928-931, 1977.

403. Q. Name the most common musculoskeletal "trigger points" in the fibrositis syndrome.

A. Although there may be many "trigger points," the most typical locations are as follows: the midpoint of the upper border of the trapezius, the extensor muscles slightly distal to the lateral epicondyle, the second costochondral junction, the fat pad medial to the knee, along the intervertebral ligaments at L4 to S1 and C4 to C6, medial border of the scapula, and the upper outer quadrant of the buttock.

REF: Smythe, H.A. and Moldofsky, H. "Two contributions to understanding of the "fibrositis" syndrome." Bull Rheum Dis 18:1, 928-931, 1977.

404. Q. Discuss the sleep disturbances that are common to patients with fibrositis.

A. In general, patients with fibrositis have a variety of sleep disturbances and often awaken with intensification of pain and increased muscular stiffness and fatigue. Although no alteration of rapid eye movement (REM) sleep was found, a characteristic pattern of alpha wave intrusion superimposed upon the slow wave (delta) rhythm was frequently present in patients with the fibrositis syndrome.

REF: Smythe, H.A. and Moldofsky, H. "Two contributions to understanding of the "fibrositis" syndrome." Bull Rheum Dis 18:1, 928-931, 1977.

405. Q. What is the potential role of hydroxyapatite crystals in the exacerbation of joint disease in degenerative osteoarthritis?

A. Hydroxyapatite crystals have now been identified within synovial fluid where they are localized to vacuoles within mononuclear cells. Light microscopy reveals them to be purplish staining cytoplasmic inclusions or extracellular globules. Occasionally they may resemble uric acid or

calicum pyrophosphate crystals and appear birefringent.
It has been hypothesized that these crystals may produce a
crystal induced acute synovitis analogous to that which may
be seen with uric acid and calcium pyrophosphate crystal
deposition disease. Injection of hydroxyapatite crystals into
the knee joints of dogs indeed results in acute synovitis.

REF: Schumacher, H.R., Smolyo, A.P., Tse, R.L., and
Maurer, K. "Arthritis associated with apatite crystals."
Ann Intern Med 87, 411-416, 1977.

406. Q. What is Lyme arthritis, which has recently been
described in Connecticut?

A. This is a recently described inflammatory arthritis which appears to be due to an arthropod vector. Its
name derives from the geographical location where most of
the cases have originated, Old Lyme, Lyme, and East
Haddam, which are three contiguous communities in
Connecticut. Erythema chronicum migrans is a skin condition which typically precedes the development of an oligoarticular or monoarticular arthritis most often affecting
the knees. Symptoms last a week or so, but on occasion
may persist for months. Neurologic manifestations, myocardial conduction defects, elevated sedimentation rates,
and elevated serum IgM levels may also be found.

REF: Steere, A.C., Malawista, S.E., Hardin, J.A., et.al.
Ann Intern Med 86, 685-698, 1977.

407. Q. Describe the radiographic features of hyperparathyroidism on the bony skeleton.

A. Whether it is primary hyperparathyroidism or
secondary disease as might be seen in renal insufficiency,
the primary event in hyperparathyroidism is osseous resorption. The typical radiographic features include sub-
periosteal bone resportion and subchondral resorption especially at the acromioclavicular, sternoclavicular and
sacroiliac joints and symphysis pubis, which may simulate
the findings seen in ankylosing spondylitis. In secondary
hyperparathyroidism due to renal failure, soft tissue

calcification and vascular calcification are not infrequently
present.

REF: Resnick, D. "Disorders of the axial skeleton which
are lesser known, poorly recognized or misunderstood."
Bull Rheum Dis 28:2,3, 932-939, 1977-78.

BY QUESTION NUMBER

Other Books Available

NURSING EXAM REVIEW BOOKS

501	Vol.	1	Medical-Surgical Nursing	$ 5.00
502	Vol.	2	Psychiatric-Mental Health Nursing	5.00
503	Vol.	3	Maternal-Child Health Nursing	5.00
504	Vol.	4	Basic Sciences	5.00
505	Vol.	5	Anatomy and Physiology	5.00
506	Vol.	6	Pharmacology	5.00
507	Vol.	7	Microbiology	5.00
508	Vol.	8	Nutrition & Diet Therapy	5.00
509	Vol.	9	Community Health	5.00
510	Vol.	10	History and Law of Nursing	5.00
511	Vol.	11	Fundamentals of Nursing	5.00
711			Practical Nursing Exam. Review — Vol. 1	5.00

NURSING OUTLINE SERIES

374	Cancer Nursing	$ 8.00
382	Community Health Nursing	6.00
384	Critical Care Nursing	
392	Gastroenterology Nursing	
388	Gynecologic Nursing	
377	Maternity Nursing	6.00
378	Nursing Fundamentals	6.00
375	Nutrition in Nursing	6.00
381	Orthopedic Nursing	6.00
379	Psychiatric-Mental Health Nursing	6.00

NURSING SELF-ASSESSMENT BOOKS

288	S.A.C.K. in Cardiopulmonary Nursing	$ 8.00
292	S.A.C.K. in Child Health Nursing	8.00
285	S.A.C.K. in Community Health Nursing	8.00
295	S.A.C.K. in Geriatric Nursing	8.00
299	S.A.C.K. in Maternity Nursing	8.00
243	S.A.C.K. in Neurology & Neurosurgical Nursing	8.00
715	S.A.C.K. for the Nurse Anesthetist	8.50

NURSING CASE STUDY BOOKS

036	Maternity Nursing Case Studies	$ 8.50
391	Psych. Comm. Mental Health Nrsg. Case St.	8.50

MODERN NURSING SERIES

861	Neurology for Nurses	$ 4.00
855	A Handbook for Nurses	4.00
862	The Nursing of Accidents	4.00
866	Emergency and Acute Care	4.00
867	Venereology for Nurses	4.00
868	The Management & Nursing of Burns	4.00
857	Microbiology in Modern Nursing	4.00
856	Obstetrics & Gynecology for Nurses	4.00
858	The Older Patient, An Introduction to Geriatrics	
863	Principles of Medicine & Med. Nursing	4.00
864	Principles of Surgery & Surgery Nursing	4.00
865	Psychology & Psychiatry for Nurses	4.00
859	Communicable Diseases	4.00

OTHER BOOKS FOR NURSES

968	Ambulatory Care Nursing Procedure & Empl. Hlth. Svc. Manual	$12.00
869	Nephrology for Nurses	8.50
376	Nursing and the Nephrology Patient	8.50
358	Renal Transplantation — A Nursing Perspective	8.50

NURSING ESSAY Q & A REVIEW BOOKS

371	Emergency & Disaster Nursing Cont. Ed. Rev.	$ 8.00
373	Gastroenterology Nursing Continuing Ed. Rev.	8.00
399	Intensive Care Nursing Continuing Ed. Review	6.00
357	Neurology & Neurosurg. Nrsg. Cont. Ed. Rev.	8.00
356	Nurse Anesthetists Continuing Ed. Review	10.00
350	Obstetric Nursing Continuing Ed. Review	8.00
397	Orthopedic & Rehab. Nursing Cont. Educ. Rev.	8.00
361	Pediatric Nursing Continuing Ed. Review	8.00
351	Psychiatric-Mental Health Nrsg. Cont. Ed. Rev.	8.00
396	Respiratory Nursing Continuing Ed. Review	8.00

ALLIED HEALTH REVIEW BOOKS

411	Medical State Board Review — Basic Sciences	$12.00
412	Medical State Board Review — Clinical Sciences	12.00
473	Cardiopulm. Techn. Exam. Review — Vol. 1	8.50
454	Cytology Exam. Review Book — Vol. 1	8.50
367	Cytology E.R.B. — Vol. 2 (Essay Q & A)	8.50
431	Dental Exam. Review Book — Vol. 1	12.00
432	Dental Exam. Review Book — Vol. 2	12.00
433	Dental Exam. Review Book — Vol. 3	12.00
461	Dental Hygiene Exam. Review — Vol. 1	8.50
465	Emergency Med. Techn. Exam. Rev. — Vol. 1	8.50
466	Emergency Med. Techn. Exam. Rev. — Vol. 2	8.50
424	Immunology Exam. Review Book — Vol. 1	12.00
455	Laboratory Assistants Exam. Rev. Bk. — Vol. 1	8.50
490	Medical Assistants Exam. Rev. Bk. — Vol. 1	8.50
495	Medical Librarian Exam. Rev. Bk. — Vol. 1	8.50
369	Medical Records Administration Cont. Ed. Rev.	12.00
496	Medical Record Library Science — Vol. 1	8.50
451	Medical Technology Exam. Review — Vol. 1	8.50
452	Medical Technology Exam. Review — Vol. 2	8.50
331	Nuclear Medicine Technology Cont. Ed. Rev.	12.00
457	Nuclear Medicine Technology Exam. Rev. Book.	12.00
475	Occupational Therapy Exam. Review — Vol. 1	8.50
469	Optometry Exam. Review — Vol. 1	12.00
470	Optometry Exam. Review — Vol. 2	12.00
421	Pharmacy Exam. Review Book — Vol. 1	8.50
430	Mill's Pharmacy State Board Q & A	12.00
481	Physical Therapy Exam. Review — Vol. 1	8.50
482	Physical Therapy Exam. Review — Vol. 2	8.50
487	Radiobiology Exam. Review Book	8.50
471	Respiratory Therapy Exam. Review — Vol. 1	8.50
344	Respiratory Therapy Exam. Review — Vol. 2	8.50
423	Sanitarian's Examination Review Book	12.00
441	X-Ray Technology Exam. Review — Vol. 1	8.50
442	X-Ray Technology Exam. Review — Vol. 2	8.50
443	X-Ray Technology Exam. Review — Vol. 3	8.50

TYPIST HANDBOOKS

976	Medical Typist's Guide for Hx & Physicals	$ 6.00
981	Radiology Typist Handbook	6.00
991	Surgical Typist Handbook	6.00
973	Transcribers Guide to Medical Terminology	6.00

LANGUAGE GUIDES

721	English-Spanish Guide for Medical Personnel	$ 3.00
961	Multilingual Guide for Medical Personnel	4.00
722	Spanish for Hospital Personnel	3.00

Prices subject to change.

P

Other Books Available

MEDICAL EXAM REVIEW BOOKS

101	Vol. 1	Comprehensive	$15.00
102	Vol. 2	Clinical Medicine	8.50
123	Vol. 2A	Txtbk. Study Guide Internal Medicine	8.50
130	Vol. 2B	Txtbk. Study Guide Internal Medicine	8.50
153	Vol. 2C	Txtbk. Study Guide of Cardiology	8.50
103	Vol. 3	Basic Sciences	8.50
104	Vol. 4	Obstetrics-Gynecology	8.50
152	Vol. 4A	Txtbk. Study Guide of Gynecology	8.50
105	Vol. 5	Surgery	8.50
150	Vol. 5A	Txtbk. Study Guide of Surgery	8.50
106	Vol. 6	Public Health & Preventive Medicine	8.50
107	Vol. 7	Psychiatry	8.50
156	Vol. 7A	Txtbk. Study Guide of Psychiatry	8.50
108	Vol. 8	Neurology	8.50
111	Vol. 11	Pediatrics	8.50
157	Vol. 11A	Txtbk. Study Guide of Pediatrics	8.50
112	Vol. 12	Anesthesiology	8.50
113	Vol. 13	Orthopaedics	15.00
114	Vol. 14	Urology	15.00
115	Vol. 15	Ophthalmology	15.00
116	Vol. 16	Otolaryngology	15.00
117	Vol. 17	Radiology	15.00
118	Vol. 18	Thoracic Surgery	15.00
119	Vol. 19	Neurological Surgery	15.00
128	Vol. 20	Physical Medicine	15.00
127	Vol. 21	Dermatology	15.00
141	Vol. 22	Gastroenterology	15.00
126	Vol. 23	Child Psychiatry	15.00
143	Vol. 24	Pulmonary Diseases	15.00
133	Vol. 25	Nuclear Medicine	15.00
132	Vol. 26	Allergy	15.00
129	Vol. 27	Plastic Surgery	18.00
138	Vol. 28	Cardiovascular Diseases	15.00
146	Vol. 29	Oncology	15.00
147	Vol. 30	Infectious Diseases	15.00
144	Vol. 31	Rheumatology	15.00
148	Vol. 32	Hematology	15.00
131	Vol. 33	Endocrinology	15.00
176	Vol. 34	Nephrology	15.00
175	Vol. 35	Pediatric Neurology	15.00
179	Vol. 36	Trauma Surgery	15.00
120	ECFMG	Exam Review — Part One	9.00
121	ECFMG	Exam Review — Part Two	9.00

BASIC SCIENCE REVIEW BOOKS

201	Anatomy Review	$ 8.00
202	Biochemistry Review	8.00
215	Digestive System Basic Sciences	8.00
207	Embryology Review	8.00
220	Gross Anatomy Review	8.00
222	Head and Neck Anatomy Review	8.00
212	Heart & Vascular Systems Basic Sciences	10.00
219	Histology Review	8.00
203	Microbiology Review	8.00
210	Nervous System Basic Sciences	10.00
218	Neuroanatomy Review	8.00
204	Pathology Review	8.00
205	Pharmacology Review	8.00
206	Physiology Review	8.00
213	Respiratory System Basic Sciences	10.00
214	Urinary System Basic Sciences	10.00
155	Medical Physiology Textbook Study Guide	8.00

MEDICAL OUTLINE SERIES

631	Cancer Chemotherapy	$12.00
630	Supplement to Cancer Chemotherapy	3.00
613	Child Psychiatry	12.00
710	Diabetes — A Clinical Guide	12.00
614	Endocrinology	12.00
628	General Pathology	12.00
662	Histology	10.00
667	Musculoskeletal System	12.00
671	Neonatology	12.00
622	Nephrology	14.00
664	Orthopedic Surgery	12.00
661	Otolaryngology	12.00
624	Pediatric Allergy	12.00
674	Pediatric Endocrinology	14.00
659	Pediatric Infectious Diseases	
658	Pediatric Radiology	15.00
621	Psychiatry	10.00
619	Traumatic Surgery	12.00
611	Urology	12.00

NEW DIRECTIONS IN THERAPY SERIES

678	Endocrinology	$12.00
682	Hematologic Diseases	12.00

SPECIALTY BOARD REVIEW BOOKS

314	Cardiology Specialty Board Review	$15.00
311	Dermatology Specialty Board Review	15.00
309	Family Practice Specialty Board Review	15.00
316	Gastroenterology Specialty Board Review	15.00
303	Internal Medicine Specialty Board Review	15.00
306	Neurology Specialty Board Review	15.00
304	Obstetrics-Gynecology Specialty Board Review	15.00
305	Pathology Specialty Board Review	15.00
301	Pediatrics Specialty Board Review	15.00
312	Psychiatry Specialty Board Review	15.00
302	Surgery Specialty Board Review	15.00
313	Essential Otolaryngology	18.00
307	The Psychiatry Boards	15.00

CASE STUDY BOOKS

027	Allergy Case Studies	$12.00
070	Arrhythmias Case Studies	
001	Cardiology Case Studies	12.00
012	Chest Diseases Case Studies	12.00
062	Child Abuse and Neglect Case Studies	12.00
029	Child Psychiatry Case Studies	12.00
014	Cutaneous Medicine Case Studies	9.00
031	Diabetes Mellitus Case Studies	12.00
003	ECG Case Studies	9.00
040	Echocardiography Case Studies	12.00
008	Endocrinology Case Studies	12.00
005	Gynecologic Oncology Case Studies	
020	Hematology Case Studies	12.00
011	Infectious Diseases Case Studies	12.00
022	Kidney Disease Case Studies	12.00
006	Neurology Case Studies	12.00
046	Neuropathology Case Studies	15.00
037	Neuroradiology Case Studies	15.00
034	Occupational Therapy Case Studies	12.00
030	Orthopedic Surgery Case Studies	12.00
021	Otolaryngology Case Studies	12.00
042	Pediatric Anesthesia Case Studies	12.00
018	Pediatric Hematology Case Studies	12.00
007	Pediatric Neurology Case Studies	18.00
023	Pediatric Oculo-Neural Diseases Case Studies	12.00
033	Pediatric Oncology Case Studies	15.00
064	Pediatric Radiology Case Studies	15.00
069	Pediatric Surgery Case Studies	
043	Perinatology Case Studies	18.00
015	Renal Transplantation Case Studies	12.00
019	Respiratory Care Case Studies	12.00
063	Surgical Oncology Case Studies	16.00
068	Surgical Pathology Case Studies	
038	Thyroid Case Studies	12.00
017	Urology Case Studies	12.00
026	X-Ray Case Studies	12.00

PATHOLOGY AND PATHOPHYSIOLOGY

CASE STUDIES SERIES

075	Cardiopulmonary	$12.00
076	Hematologic & Reticuloendothelial	12.00
077	Renal, Genitourinary & Breast	12.00
078	Digestive & Hepatobiliary	12.00
079	Endocrine	12.00
080	Central Nervous System & Neuromuscular	12.00

PRACTITIONERS GUIDES

720	Dermatology	$12.00
705	E.N.T. Disorders	12.00
709	Hypertension	12.00
704	OB-Gynecology Disorders	12.00
703	Ophthalmologic Disorders	12.00
712	Pediatric Neurology	12.00
713	Physical Medicine & Rehabilitation	12.00

DISCUSSIONS IN PATIENT MANAGEMENT SERIES

878	Acute Renal Failure	$ 8.00
887	Ankylosing Spondylitis	
876	Asthma	8.00
891	Bleeding Disorders	
888	Gout and Pseudogout	
898	Hypothyroidism	
880	Infectious & Parasitic Diseases of the Intestine	8.00
895	Nephrotic Syndrome	
879	Peptic Ulcer	

FOCUS ON CLINICAL DIAGNOSIS SERIES

825	Nuclear Medicine	$12.00
826	Pediatric Allergic Diseases	12.00

Other Books Available

PRACTICAL POINTS BOOKS

731	in Allergy	$12.00
700	in Anesthesiology	12.00
733	in Gastroenterology	12.00
702	in Pediatrics	12.00
724	in Pulmonary Diseases	12.00

SELF-ASSESSMENT BOOKS

296	Self-Assess. of Current Knowledge in Allergy	$12.00
245	S.A.C.K. in Anesthesiology	12.00
289	S.A.C.K. in Blood Banking	8.50
276	S.A.C.K. in Cardiothoracic Surgery	12.00
275	S.A.C.K. in Cardiovascular Disease	12.00
287	S.A.C.K. in Child Psychiatry	12.00
266	S.A.C.K. in Clinical Biochemistry	8.50
297	S.A.C.K. in Clin. Endo., Metab. & Diab.	12.00
281	S.A.C.K. in Clinical Pharmacy	8.50
278	S.A.C.K. in Diagnostic Radiology	12.00
261	S.A.C.K. in Family Practice	12.00
235	S.A.C.K. in Forensic and Organic Psychiatry	
178	S.A.C.K. in Forensic Pathology & Legal Medicine	12.00
248	S.A.C.K. in Hematology, Part 1 – Textbk. Rev.	14.00
283	S.A.C.K. in Hematology, Part 2 – Lit. Review.	12.00
263	S.A.C.K. in Infectious Diseases	12.00
257	S.A.C.K. in Internal Medicine	12.00
273	S.A.C.K. in Medical Technology – Hematology	8.50
240	S.A.C.K. in Neonatology	12.00
280	S.A.C.K. in Nephrology	12.00
247	S.A.C.K. in Neurological Surgery	15.00
254	S.A.C.K. in Neurology	12.00
239	S.A.C.K. in Nuclear Medicine	12.00
260	S.A.C.K. in Obstetrics & Gynecology	12.00
249	S.A.C.K. in Occupational Therapy	8.50
284	S.A.C.K. in Oncology	12.00
474	S.A.C.K. for the Operating Room Technician	8.50
255	S.A.C.K. in Ophthalmology	15.00
244	S.A.C.K. in Orthodontics	12.00
270	S.A.C.K. in Otolaryngology	12.00
253	S.A.C.K. in Pathology	12.00
256	S.A.C.K. in Pediatrics	12.00
241	S.A.C.K. in Pediatric Cardiology	12.00
277	S.A.C.K. in Pediatric Hematology & Oncology	12.00
272	S.A.C.K. in Pharmacy	8.50
252	S.A.C.K. in Psychiatry	12.00
271	S.A.C.K. in Pulmonary Diseases	12.00
274	S.A.C.K. in Radiologic Technology	8.50
258	S.A.C.K. in Rheumatology	12.00
250	S.A.C.K. in Surgery	12.00
259	S.A.C.K. in Surgery for Family Physicians	12.00
286	S.A.C.K. in Therapeutic Radiology	12.00
251	S.A.C.K. in Urology	12.00

ESSAY Q. & A. REVIEW BOOKS

353	Anesthesiology Cont. Education Review	$12.00
339	Blood Banking Principles Review Book	10.00
337	Cardiology Review	12.00
364	Cardiovascular Disease Contg. Ed. Review	12.00
343	Child & Adolescent Psychiatry Cont. Ed. Rev.	12.00
338	Colon & Rectal Surgery Cont. Educ. Review	12.00
341	Dermatology Continuing Education Review	12.00
362	Diabetes & Metab. Disorders Cont. Ed. Rev.	12.00
372	Diagnostic Radiology Continuing Ed. Review	12.00
345	Neurology Continuing Education Review	12.00
347	Ophthalmology Review	12.00
349	Orthopedics Review	12.00
342	Pediatrics Continuing Education Review	12.00
360	Pediatric Hematol. & Oncology Cont. Ed. Rev.	12.00
332	Pediatric Surgery Continuing Education Review	12.00
335	Physical Medicine & Rehabilitation Continuing Education Review	12.00
354	Plastic Surgery Continuing Education Review	12.00
352	Psychiatry Continuing Education Review	12.00
346	Therapeutic Radiology Continuing Ed. Review	12.00

JOURNAL ARTICLE COMPILATIONS

795	Emergency Room Journal Articles	$12.00
799	Hospital Pharmacy Journal Articles	12.00
530	Medical Psychiatry Journal Articles	12.00
797	Outpatient Services Journal Articles, 2nd Ed.	12.00
792	PSRO Journal Articles	18.00
523	Selected Papers in Inhalation Therapy	12.00

OTHER BOOKS

601	Acid Base Homeostasis	$ 5.00
326	Annual Review of Allergy 1973	15.00
327	Annual Review of Allergy 1974	15.00
328	Annual Review of Allergy 1975/76	18.00
979	Atlas of C.T. Scans in Pediatric Neurology	36.00
900	Bailey & Love's Short Practice of Surgery	48.00
978	Basic Correlative Echocardiography Technique and Interpretation	16.00
932	Benign & Malignant Bladder Tumors	18.00
652	Blood Bank Policies & Procedures	12.00
860	Blood Groups	5.00
759	Cerebral Degenerations in Childhood	10.00
730	Clinical Diagnostic Pearls	6.00
602	Concentrations of Solutions	5.00
983	Critical Care Manual	16.00
754	Cryogenics in Surgery	36.00
675	Curr. Concepts Breast Canc. & Tumor Immunol.	18.00
677	Curr. Concepts in Intra-Abdominal Cancers	18.00
745	Current Therapy of Allergy	18.00
748	Diagnosis & Treatment of Breast Lesions	18.00
974	Dynamics of Dental Practice Administration	18.00
987	Echocardiography – A Manual for Technicians	14.00
984	Emergency Care Manual	8.50
740	Essential Neurology	
603	Fundamental Orthopedics	6.00
758	Fundamentals of Homeostasis	8.50
992	Fundamentals of Operating Room Technology	
962	Guide to Medical Reports	4.50
985	Guide to Patient Evaluation	10.00
982	Human Anatomical Terminology	4.00
919	Illustrated Laboratory Techniques	12.00
753	Introduction to Acupuncture Anesthesia	6.00
975	Introduction to Blood Banking	10.00
729	Introduction to the Clinical History	4.00
965	Laboratory Diagnosis of Infectious Disease	8.50
995	Malpractice Made Easy	15.00
964	Math for Med Techs	8.00
942	Medallion World Atlas	34.95
990	Medical Glossaround	3.00
242	Microbiology & Immunology – A Positive Statement Manual	8.50
736	Neoplasms of the Gastrointestinal Tract	24.00
600	Neurophysiology Study Guide	8.00
752	Outpatient Hemorrhoidectomy Ligation Techn.	15.00
993	Pacemaker & Valve Identification Guide	40.00
050	Pediatrics – A Problem-Oriented Approach	8.50
422	Physician's Assistant Exam. Review Book	12.00
986	Primary Care of Young Adults – A Practitioner's Manual	12.00
963	Profiles in Surgery, Gynecology & Obstetrics	6.00
966	The Radioactive Patient	12.00
486	Radiological Physics Examination Review	12.00
744	Skin, Heredity & Malignant Neoplasms	24.00
967	Teaching the Retarded Child	9.00
743	Testicular Tumors	30.00
756	Tissue Adhesives in Surgery	30.00
977	Understanding Hematology	10.00
832	Wall Atlas of Human Anatomy	130.00

MEDICAL HANDBOOKS

648	Child Abuse and Neglect Handbook	$12.00
610	Clinical Nuclear Medicine	12.00
639	E.N.T. Emergencies	10.00
632	General Surgical Emergencies	10.00
640	Gynecologic Emergencies	10.00
635	Medical Emergencies	10.00
643	Neurologic Emergencies	10.00
604	Neurology	10.00
634	Obstetric Emergencies	10.00
633	Ophthalmologic Emergencies	12.00
637	Pediatric Anesthesia	10.00
636	Pediatric Neurology	18.00
649	Pediatric Respiratory Intensive Care Handbook	12.00
642	Pediatric Surgical Emergencies	12.00
645	Psychiatric Emergencies	12.00
647	Urologic Emergencies	10.00